PREVENTION, DETECTION AND MANAGEMENT OF ORAL CANCER

Edited by **Sivapatham Sundaresan**

Prevention, Detection and Management of Oral Cancer
http://dx.doi.org/10.5772/intechopen.79314
Edited by Sivapatham Sundaresan

Contributors

Zahra Al Timimi, Mohammed Saleem Ismail Alhabeel, A. Hameed Khan, Nihat Akbulut, Ahmet Altan, Neeti Kapre, Monica Mahajan, Apeksha Hore, Masakatsu Fukuda, Hideaki Sakashita, Sivapatham Sundaresan

Notice

Statements and opinions expressed in the chapters are these of the individual contributors and not necessarily those of the editors or publisher. No responsibility is accepted for the accuracy of information contained in the published chapters. The publisher assumes no responsibility for any damage or injury to persons or property arising out of the use of any materials, instructions, methods or ideas contained in the book.

First published in London, United Kingdom, 2019 by IntechOpen
IntechOpen is the global imprint of INTECHOPEN LIMITED, registered in England and Wales, registration number: 11086078, 7th floor, 10 Lower Thames Street, London,
EC3R 6AF, United Kingdom
Printed in Croatia

British Library Cataloguing-in-Publication Data
A catalogue record for this book is available from the British Library

Additional hard and PDF copies can be obtained from orders@intechopen.com

Prevention, Detection and Management of Oral Cancer, Edited by Sivapatham Sundaresan
p. cm.
Print ISBN 978-1-78984-502-0
Online ISBN 978-1-78984-503-7
eBook (PDF) ISBN 978-1-78984-604-1

For EU product safety concerns:
IN TECH d.o.o., Prolaz Marije Krucifikse Kozulić 3, 51000 Rijeka, Croatia,
info@intechopen.com or visit our website at intechopen.com.

Meet the editor

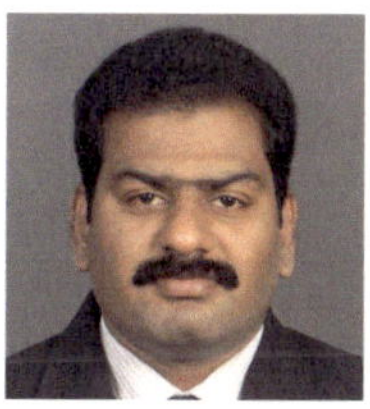

Assosiate Professor, Dr. Sundaresan received his M. Phil. in Biochemistry in 1999 from Annamalai University and his Ph.D. in Biochemistry in 2003 from Annamalai University as well. He currently teaches research methodology at SRM MCH and RC. Dr. Sundaresan is Ph.D guide in Medical and Health sciences, and is also incharge for the Central Research Laboratory. He is a Journal editorial board member and reviewer for many national and international publications. He is a member of the Association of Clinical Biochemists of India (ACBI), member of the Society of Biological Chemists –MSBC and member of Indian Inborn Errors of Metabolism society IB.

Contents

Preface

Oral cancer is frequently diagnosed late, when the disease has advanced with lesions that are large and deeply invasive and with metastasis to regional lymph nodes, leading to increased mortality. Moreover, late diagnosis and treatment often result in considerable morbidity of oral and maxillofacial structures and poor appearance and function following therapy. Incidence of cancer in the country has been increasing over the last few decades. This book covers the topic of oral cancer in a concise but detailed manner. The book certainly achieves its aim: enhancing knowledge of the many aspects of care and management that oral cancer encompasses. The opening chapter presents the pathogenesis of cancer by introducing the reader to the cellular, histological, and molecular changes that occur in the disease process. This is followed by detailed chapters on different, newer aspects of oral cancer, which will enrich all clinicians who aim to promote preventive advice. Overall, the book fulfills its purpose entirely in updating researchers on oral cancer.

This book will help researchers and clinicians in understanding the fundamentals and management of oral cancer in individual patients.

Dr. S. Sundaresan M.Sc., M.Phil., Ph.D.
Associate Professor
Department of Medical Reserch
SRM Institute of Science and Technology
India

Chapter 1

Introductory Chapter: Head and Neck Cancer

Sivapatham Sundaresan and Paliarasu Rajapriya

Additional information is available at the end of the chapter

http://dx.doi.org/10.5772/intechopen.86272

1. Introduction

Cancer is the major cause of mortality in economically advanced nations, and in developing nations it is the second leading cause of death [1]. The survival rate due to the heterogeneity in treatment offered within centers across India for buccal mucosa cancer in India is 5 years ranges from 60 to 80% for stage I disease to 5 to 15% for locally progressive disease [2, 3].

Squamous cell carcinoma (HNSCC) develops in the oral cavity, larynx, or hypopharynx and oropharynx. In accordance with incidence rate, it is reported as the sixth leading cancer worldwide [4]. It is likely that approximately 600,000 cases have been established worldwide, and the 5-year survival rate is only 40–50% in patients with HNSCC [5]. In a 5-year period, estimated new cases of head and neck cancer were 300,000 and approximately 145,000 deaths in 2012 and 702,000 predominant cases [6]. It was reported that two-thirds of the global incidence of oral cancer occurs in low- and middle-income countries (LMICs). In that, half of those cases are in South Asia. In India alone, one-fifth of the population have head and neck cancer and one-fourth of all head and neck cancer demises [6]. **Figure 1** illustrates the region of all head and neck cancers.

2. Pathogenesis of head and neck cancer

There is a prolonged preclinical phase for head and neck cancer, and also it constitutes well-documented precancerous lesions. The precancerous lesions comprise leukoplakia, erythroplakia, oral submucous fibrosis (OSMF), lichen planus, and chronic traumatic ulcers. The frequency at annual rate was estimated to be in the range from 0.13 to 2.2% during the transformation of oral precancerous lesions to cancer [7, 8].

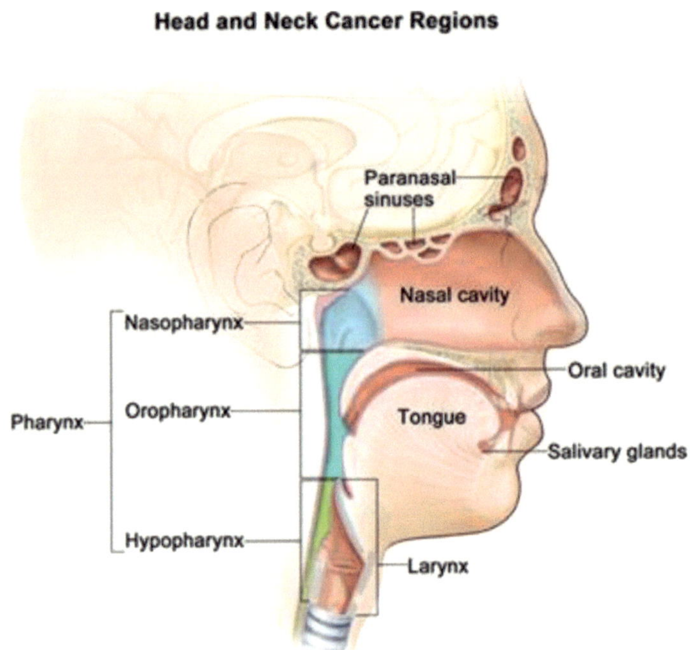

Figure 1. Head and Neck Cancer Regions.

The clinical conditions such as nodular lesions, painless small ulcers, or growths present in very early preclinical invasive early stage cancers culminate the disease. Changes can be easily seen and are clinically detectable through careful visual inspection, and palpation of the oral mucosa was the hallmark of processes. Highlighting the disease prognosis that localized early head and neck cancers ˂4 cm that has not spread to the regional lymph nodes can be successfully treated with either radiotherapy or surgery resulting in 80% of 5-year survival rates [9].

Leukoplakia may be clinically categorized as homogeneous or nonhomogeneous condition, in which a white snowy plaque or patch will form on the tongue. If the lesions have a thin, flat, uniform, smooth, and white appearance, it is categorized as homogeneous, and nonhomogeneous lesions may have a white and red appearance or tiny, white, pinhead-size raised nodules on a reddish background or a proliferative, warty presence. Erythroplakia exists as a red patch with a smooth or granular surface that cannot be categorized clinically or pathologically as any other definable disease [10]. Erythroplakia has a higher chance than leukoplakia to anchorage occult invasive cancer and to undergo malignant transformation.

Interweaving white lines (known as *Wickham's striae*) with a reddish border or as a mix of reddish and ulcerated areas will appear on oral lichen planus. OSMF, mostly restricted to the people of Indian subcontinent origin and in certain Pacific islands such as the Mariana Islands, presents with a blanching of the oral mucosa, burning sensation, and intolerance to spicy food. As the disease progresses, hardening and weaken of the oral and pharyngeal mucosa occur, leading to reduced mouth opening and difficulty in swallowing and speaking. Smokers who smoke with the lighted end of the tobacco product inside the mouth, known as reverse smoking, will be acquired with palatal lesions resulting in white or mixed reddish-white lesions of the palate [10].

A higher risk of malignant alteration may be related with the factors like female gender, lesions of long period, large precancerous lesions, precancerous lesions in nonusers of tobacco, tongue, and floor of mouth lesions, nonhomogeneous lesions, and lesions showing epithelial dysplasia and aneuploidy [11]. However, during the follow-up in patients, it is impossible to predict with certainty where the precancerous lesion will become malignant. The malignant alteration of precancerous lesions can be prevented by interventions, such as avoiding the use of tobacco and consuming alcohol and by excision of the lesions in selected cases.

3. Incidence and mortality

WHO conveyed that head and neck cancer occurrence and death are high in India, Papua New Guinea, and Taiwan, China, where the habit of chewing betel quid's with tobacco or without tobacco or areca nut chewing is common, as well as in France, Eastern Europe, and parts of South America such as Brazil and Uruguay, where tobacco smoking and alcohol ingestion are high. The age-standardized incidence rates for men are, on average, twice as high as those for women. WHO reported that in selected countries where some reliable cancer registries exist, India is highest and Belarus is lowest, with incidence rates changing by more than five times in men and women. The estimated age-standardized incidence rates of head and neck cancer also fluctuate among countries in different regions [6].

In South and Southeast Asia, buccal (cheek) mucosa is the most common site for head and neck cancer; the tongue is the most prominent site in all other regions [12]. Regional differences in frequency and the site of occurrence are related to the major causes, which are betel quid and tobacco chewing in South and Southeast Asia and alcohol and smoking in Western countries [13]. The mortality rates of head and neck cancer range between 1 and 15 per 100,000 persons in different regions; mortality rates exceed 10 per 100,000 in Eastern European countries, such as the Czech Republic, Hungary, and the Slovak Republic. Head and neck cancer mortality rates are influenced by head and neck cancer incidence, access to treatment, and deviations in site distribution.

The trends in incidence and mortality among men and women are closely correlated with the patterns and trends in tobacco and alcohol use. Increase in tobacco and areca nut chewing and alcohol consumption causes an elevated incidence rate which has been reported in Karachi [14] and in Taiwan [15]. Head and neck cancer incidence and mortality rates have been gradually falling over the past 2 decades because of declining smoking prevalence and alcohol ingestion in the US [16]. However, because of human papillomavirus (HPV), there is an increase in cancers at the base of the tongue, which has been observed in white men in the United States [17].

It was reported that over the past 2 decades, incidence and mortality rates for head and neck cancer have been declining steadily in most European countries. The increasing rates had been observed in some Central European countries, such as Hungary and the Slovak Republic, reflecting changes in alcohol and tobacco consumption [18]. There was a steady decrease in the mortality rate of head and neck cancer in France since reaching a peak in the early 1990s and the decline correlated with the reduction in alcohol consumption. Incidence and mortality have been stable in the Nordic countries, the Russian Federation, and the United Kingdom. Mortality rates have been steadily declining in Australia and Hong Kong SAR, China but increasing in Japan and the Republic of Korea [19].

4. Diet and head and neck cancer

The current report highlighted that about 15% of all cancer deaths are related to unhealthy diets, including high intake of red meat, processed meat, and sodium, as well as low intake of fruits and vegetables [20]. Most research is still not consistent about specific nutritional items yet for the cause of cancer geographically [21]. The most current comprehensive review of diet and cancer risks confirms an elevated risk related to red and processed meat but finds less evidence supporting the benefit of the consumption of fruits and vegetables in reducing risk [22]. When well-established risk factors are included in the estimation of cancer, the variations in the strength of the evidence in different studies over time makes the measurement of dietary intake problematic in epidemiological studies. Nearly 5% of cancer deaths worldwide (387,000) would be attributable to dietary risk factors [20]. Ingestion of red meat and processed meat increases the risk of colorectal cancer by an estimate of 43% [21]. Ingestion of red meat and processed meat is generally rising in low- and middle-income countries (LMICs), but is stable in high-income countries (HICs). Another major dietary risk factor is high salt intake, which increases the risk of stomach cancer. Globally, salt intake has declined, and

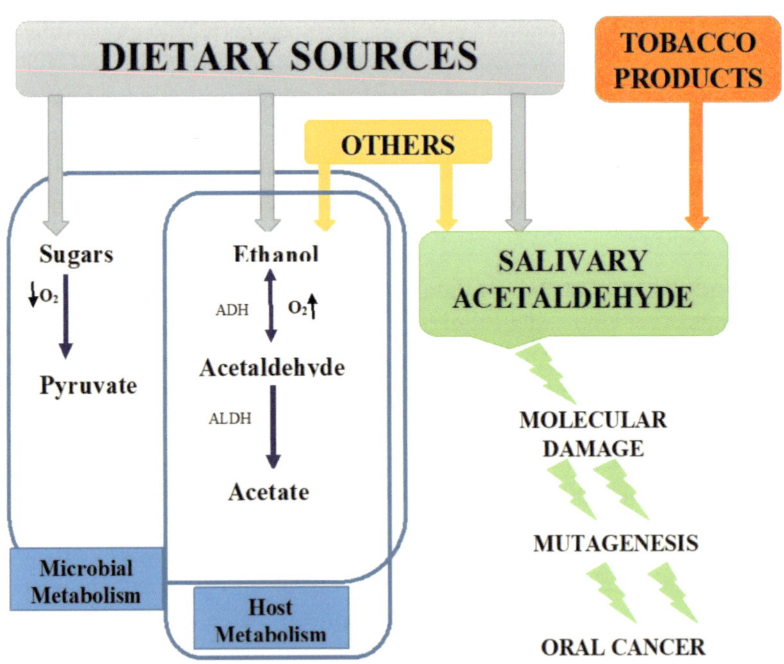

Figure 2. The mechanism of salivary involvement with diet and cancer.

the associated cancer burden has declined as a result [22]; currently, 1.5 and 2% of all cancer deaths in HICs and LMICs, respectively, are attributed to high salt intake, compared with 2.2 and 2.7%, respectively, in 1990 is highlighted by Lim and others. In the United Kingdom, 10% of new stomach cancer cases diagnosed in 2010 may be attributable to high salt intake [23].

Figure 2 describes the mechanism of salivary involvement with diet and cancer.

Over the past era, key factor in the decline in cancer incidence reported to be the better food preservation methods and reducing the salt. The levels of red meat consumption in recent decades may explain the low colorectal cancer rates in southern Asia [21], as well as the high rates in many Western European countries were reported [24, 25]. Researchers find association for obesity and overweight to cancer is firmer than the dietary evidence has been reported, indicating that 3 and 6% of cancer deaths in LMICs and HICs, respectively, can be attributed to excess weight, as quantified by the body mass index (BMI) [26, 27]. High BMI was raised as a cause of cancer deaths more substantively in LMICs, a 54% increase over the past 30 years, compared with a 26% increase in HICs over the same period [28].

5. Buccal mucosa cancer—our perspective

A buccal mucosa carcinoma is a violent form of head and neck cancer associated with the high rate of locoregional reappearance and poor existence [29]. It is the most common cancer in men and the third most common cancer in women in India [30]. National Cancer Registry Program (India) has stated approximately 13,500 cases of buccal mucosa carcinoma from various Indian cancer registries [31]. Indian Council of Medical Research guideline on buccal mucosa carcinoma management reported that there is the absence of national and international data specifically on buccal mucosa cancer, and very few randomized studies from India on various aspects of buccal mucosa cancer are available [32]. Tumor thickness and other prognostic factors were institutes to be not correct predictors of relapse and most of the studies were not adequately powered to draw a definite conclusion. Patients with head and neck cancer observed by computed tomography, magnetic resonance imaging (MRI), ultrasound-guided fine needle aspiration biopsy, and positron emission tomography (PET) have significant false positive and false negative results, invariably not capable of detecting nodal metastasis [33, 34]. Genetic alterations recognized to date have not been used clinically in the assessment of surgical margins, and no study has developed a gene signature that can accurately predict which patients with buccal cancer are at a higher risk of disease recurrence. Traditional surgical procedures may miss involved lymph nodes due to a limitation in histopathology examinations [35]. Lymph-node metastasis can be predicted by gene expression profiles of primary oral cavity squamous cell carcinomas [36]. Further, markers of prognosis will be validated by qRT-PCR technique. Gene expression profiles of primary tumor and their matched normal mucosa and comparing with different tumor stage and lymph-node status and to identify clinically significant prognostic markers is warranted.

Increase in the incidence of buccal mucosa carcinoma was observed from the hospital registry over the last 15 years [3]. The incidence and cumulative risk of buccal mucosa cancer in

Chennai were higher in both sexes among all of the states in India [37]. Currently, there are no markers that can consistently predict malignant progression in oral dysplastic lesions. Recurrent disease after surgery and radiotherapy is hard to salvage because of availability of earlier markers to predict the stage of disease [38]. It was reported that variability in the clinical course of patients remains unexplained and conventional clinicopathological parameters fail to answer all questions. Identification of novel prognostic factors may allow a rational selection of the most appropriate therapeutic options for individual patients [39].

Oral tumor thickness and other prognostic factors were found to be not correct predictors of relapse, and most of the study was not adequately powered to drought a definite conclusion. Clinicopathological parameters such as the TNM system, which are generally used as a basis for therapeutic decisions, frequently fail to predict the biologic behavior of the tumors or the patients' outcome [40]. ICMR guideline on buccal mucosa carcinoma highlights that new prognostic factors for buccal mucosa cancer are the very important need to manage it.

6. Buccal mucosa cancer and molecular markers

Estimates based on weighted averages of data from Bangalore, Mumbai, Bhopal, Chennai, and Delhi show that buccal mucosa carcinoma has an incidence of 4.0% of all malignancies in males and 3.5% of all malignancies in females. Buccal mucosa cancer is a dissimilar disease biologically, as compared to rest of head and neck cancer, and requires great care [41]. The buccal tumor was reported to differ from other tumors by early stage less often and arises from premalignant tissue with abnormal clinical appearances, which may prevent earlier diagnosis and referral from primary care [42].

Van't Veer et al. showed the ability of gene expression profiles to classify tumors into clinically appropriate groups and to predict the outcome by using supervised statistical analyses [43]. Individuals whose primary tumors bore the metastases-related gene expression program had significantly shorter survival times compared with individuals whose tumors needed it [44].

Importantly, candidate-gene approach study had reported genetic alterations in surgical resection margins in head and neck squamous cell carcinoma (HNSCC) from different disease sites, e.g., oral cavity, pharynx/hypopharynx, and larynx [45–47]. Markedly genetic alterations identified in HNSCC encompassed over-expression of eIF4E [48], TP53, and CDKN2A/P16 proteins [49].

A prognostic value with disease-free and overall survival was shown in a study of gene expression profile of three genes (GLUT3, HSAL2, and PACE4) were correlated with different clinical parameters [39]. A 4-gene signature (MMP1, COL4A1, THBS2, and P4HA2) for calculation of recurrence in OSCC had been studied in whole-genome expression profiling experiment and a meta-analysis of five microarray datasets developed [35].

Known risk factors like areca nut and betel quid reported to contain genotoxic, cytotoxic, and ability to stimulate human buccal mucosal fibroblast proliferation [50]. It was conveyed to act synergistically in the pathogenesis of oral submucous fibrosis and head and neck cancer [51].

Other risk factors such as arecoline, safrole, and nicotine, which are released in saliva during betel quid chewing plus cigarette smoking, inhibit collagen phagocytosis by fibroblast [52].

Majority of head and neck cancers are preceded by a period during which the affected epithelium shows evidence of epithelial dysplasia, although this may not always be clinically apparent [8]. Several studies have exposed great inter- and intra-examiner variability in the assessment of the presence or absence and the grade of oral epithelial dysplasia [53–56], the kappa values, in general, showing poor to a moderate bargain among examiners.

Five-year survival with single modality treatment of 19–20% was observed in patients with T3 and T4 stages [57]. Diaz and others had shown that the relapse amount was up to 45% in patients with early stage disease [58], and relapse rate in patients with nodes demanding some form of adjuvant treatment in early disease and high-risk tumors.

Mishra et al. had reported the relation between treatment failure and tumor thickness in a series of 176 patients with early buccal mucosa cancer [59]. Tumor thickness of more than 4 mm was found to be connected with lymph-node metastasis. In another study, tumor thickness of more than 5 mm was linked with nodal metastasis [60]. There are few studies described in the literature that associate the prognostic factors linked with clinical result of buccal cancer.

The molecular changes between the tumor subtypes are often accompanied by differences in clinical features, such as statistically robust differences in relapse-free and overall survival [61], and many studies found handfuls of specific genes whose expression is linked with prognosis [62].

Figure 3 demonstrates the etiopathogenesis of OSCC.

Using high-throughput analysis of multiple surgical margins and matched oral squamous cell carcinoma to classify deregulated genes with prognostic value for recurrence need to be carried out. Presence of epithelial dysplasia or tumor cells in the surgical resection margins is linked with significant risk (66%) of local recurrence [63]. However, even with histologically normal surgical margins, 10–30% of OSCC patients will still have local recurrence [64]. Gene expression profiling by high-throughput technologies has proven to be valuable tools for prediction of outcome and progression in human malignancies including head and neck cancer [65].

To impact the survival of buccal cancer patients, molecular markers must be identified, which will help target tumors with a propensity for metastatic spread. There are numerous reports on the request of molecular biological markers for the valuation of cancer risk [66]. Molecular changes in oral pre-malignancy and head and neck cancer are influenced by differences in the ethnic and etiologic characteristics in different parts of the world [67].

Despite having poor clinical risk factors, patients who need chemotherapy will have enormous potential for better individualization of treatment options in breast cancer therapy where the clinical utility of gene signatures are playing a important contribution and proved to reliably identify patients in whom adjuvant chemotherapy is certainly not indicated [68].

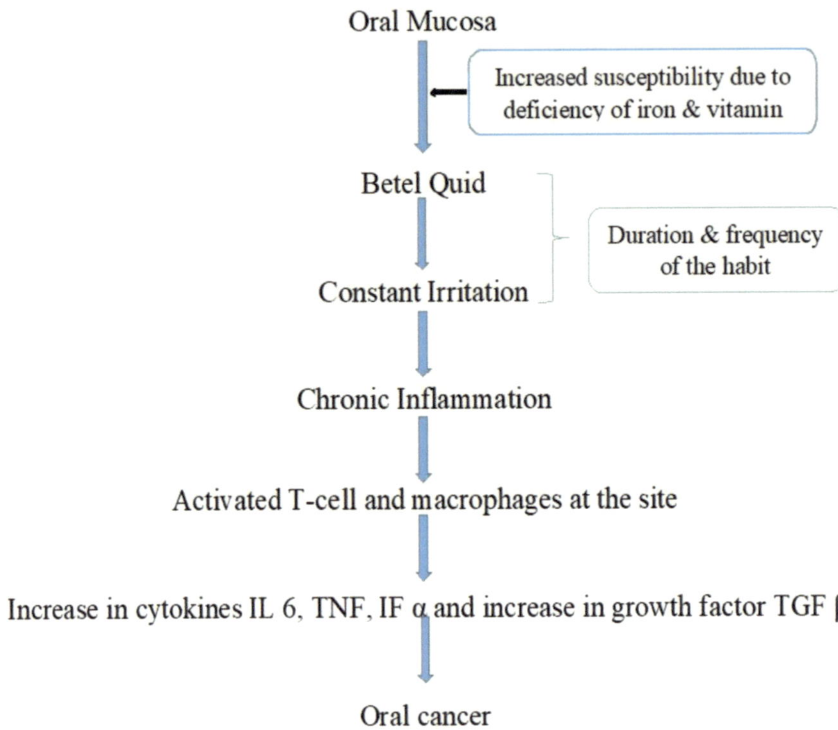

Figure 3. The etiopathogenesis of OSCC.

A specific tumor marker is not clinically available for the discovery of cancer at an early and possibly curative stage. Lymph-node metastasis is the main step in tumor progression and a risk factor for reappearance subsequent to surgery. Cluster analysis, part of data analysis of microarray, clearly parted cases with lymph-node metastasis from those without metastasis. Data indicated that sorting of patients into high- and low-risk subgroups on the basis of the prognosis summary may be useful means of guiding adjuvant therapy in patients with lymph-node positive breast cancer.

Figure 4 shows the mechanism of oral squamous carcinoma.

Patients who needed adjuvant chemotherapy but also those who did not need adjuvant chemotherapy, leading to a reduction in the number of women who would otherwise receive chemotherapy without compromising long-term clinical outcome was done using the 70-gene signature [69].

Netherlands Cancer Institute in Amsterdam (NKI) calculated expression of 70 genes was found to be statistically significantly linked with disease outcome, as defined by the presence of distant metastasis within 5 years. Metastases have also been found in the absence of clinically obvious primary tumors [70]. Ability to form distant metastases is a concern of particular method of transformation as contrasting to a selection process auxiliary the metastatic phenotype per se.

Determination of any signature genes are most important in the cascade of events driving metastasis along with tumor behavior is warranted. Bieche and others reported a 3-gene expression profile, which distinguished subgroups of patients with good, intermediate, and poor outcomes [71].

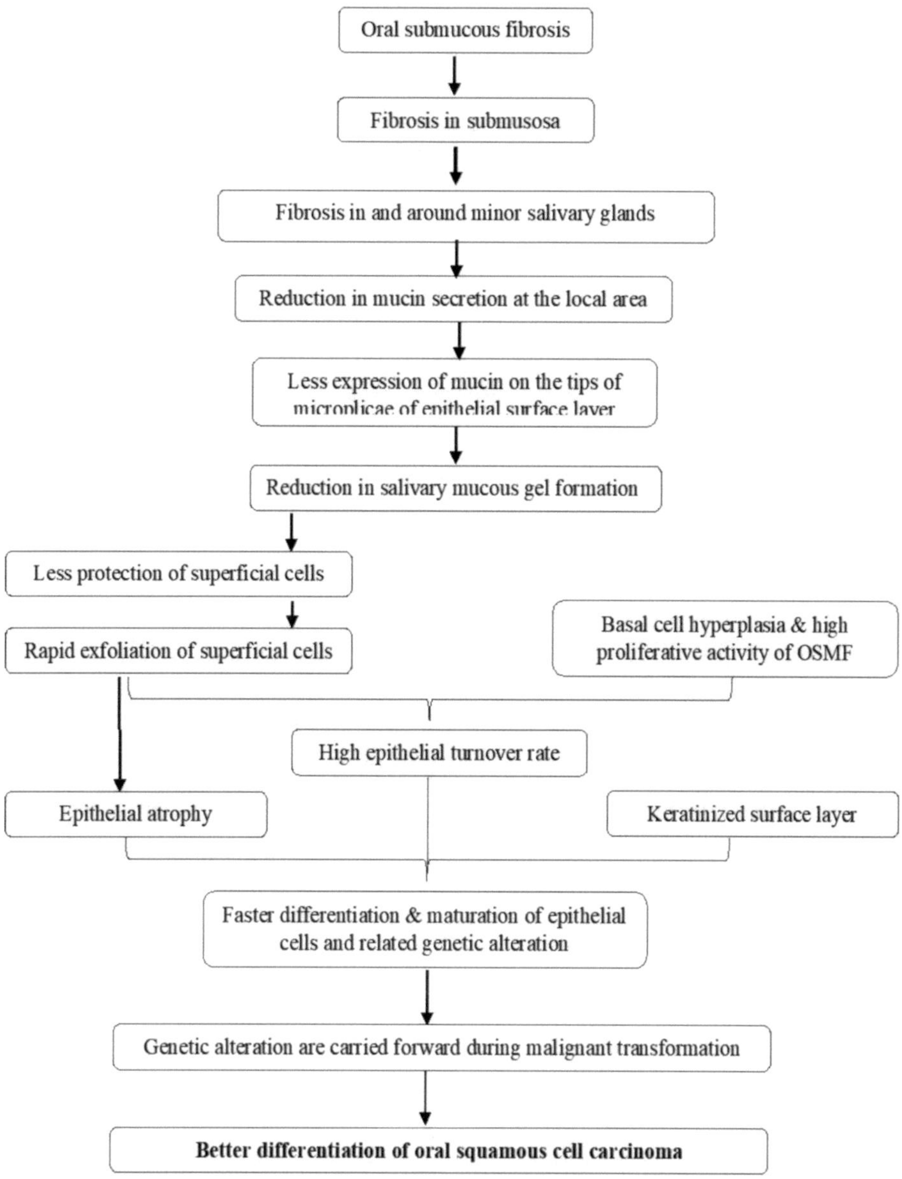

Figure 4. The mechanism of oral squamous carcinoma.

7. Head and neck cancer and research hypothesis

As the tools to categorize precancerous lesions in the mouth remain to improve, fewer men will die needlessly from head and neck cancer. Researchers are now harnessing the power of nanotechnology science to engineer strategies to investigate human fluids and tissues for abnormal molecules that are suggestive of a developing oral tumor. To detect abnormal cells and proteins in saliva that are associated with a developing oral tumor in-office diagnostic devices are being developed by investigators.

Treatment will improve, as targeted molecular therapy and personalized medicine become a truth. Predictable to guide treatment decisions for the individual patient on the basis of tumor HPV status is an evolving research, and evidence-based clinical trials are on the go. An inquiry is also defining the signaling pathways and networks that determine the development of head and neck cancer cells had been drawn, which will result in novel anticancer drugs that goals the particular molecular absences in each individual head and neck cancer patient.

Head and neck cancers are readily accessible, unlike tumors of the prostate, pancreas, or other internal organs. Rapid growth of valuable information for developing improved cure rates for both oral and other cancers is attained, and becomes more effortlessly studied cancers which may allow to accomplish the goal.

Locoregional control and overall patient survival potentially may improve the development of novel chemotherapy regimens and targeted therapeutic agents. Groups, like the Eastern Cooperative Oncology Group (ECOG), Radiation Therapy Oncology Group (RTOG), Southwest Oncology Group (SWOG), and European Organization for the Research and Treatment of Cancer (EORTC), facilitate patient enrollment into multi-institutional prospective randomized trials, which have delivered us with the necessary data to define current and future standards of care. Measures to identify biomarkers that predict disease behavior will carry on as individualized therapy evolves. Endorsed quality-of-life index measures additional define treatment results, and escalation of combined treatment likely will necessitate significant attention regarding treatment-induced toxicities is to be looked upon [72, 73]. The use of tobacco-related foodstuffs remains important worldwide, but further etiologic factors such as HPV similarly affect HNSCC presentation, behavior, and treatment [74]. Though improvement has been made throughout the past 60 years, a boundless deal remains to be consummate in head and neck cancer prevention.

Author details

Sivapatham Sundaresan* and Paliarasu Rajapriya

*Address all correspondence to: sundarbiosrm@gmail.com

Department of Medical Research, SRM MCH & RC, Kanchipuram, Tamil Nadu, India

References

[1] Ferlay J. GLOBOCAN 2008, Cancer Incidence and Mortality Worldwide: IARC Cancer Base No. 10. 2010. Avilable from: http://globocan.iarc.fr

[2] Pradhan SA. Surgery for the cancer of the buccal mucosa. Seminars in Surgical Oncology. 1989;**5**(5):318-321

[3] Iyer SG, Pradhan SA, Pai PS. Surgical treatment outcomes of localized squamous carcinoma of buccal mucosa. Head and Neck. 2004;**26**(10):897-902

[4] Kamangar F, Dores GM, Anderson WF. Patterns of cancer incidence, mortality, and prevalence across five continents: Defining priorities to reduce cancer disparities in different geographic regions of the world. Journal of Clinical Oncology. 2006;**24**(14):2137-2150

[5] Leemans CR, Braakhuis BJ, Brakenhoff RH. The molecular biology of head and neck cancer. Nature Reviews Cancer. 2011;**11**(1):9

[6] Bray F, Ren JS, Masuyer E, Ferlay J. Estimates of global cancer prevalence for 27 sites in the adult population in 2008. International Journal of Cancer. 2013;**132**(5):1133-1145

[7] Amagasa T, Yamashiro M, Uzawa N. Oral premalignant lesions: From a clinical perspective. International Journal of Clinical Oncology. 2011;**16**(1):5-14

[8] Napier SS, Speight PM. Natural history of potentially malignant oral lesions and conditions: An overview of the literature. Journal of Oral Pathology & Medicine. 2008;**37**(1):1-10

[9] Sankaranarayanan R, Ramadas K, Amarasinghe H, Subramanian S, Johnson N. Oral Cancer: Prevention, Early Detection, and Treatment. Disease Control Priorities. The World Bank, Washinton: The International Bank for Reconstruction and Development; 3rd ed; 2015. p. 85

[10] Warnakulasuriya S, Johnson NW, Van der Waal I. Nomenclature and classification of potentially malignant disorders of the oral mucosa. Journal of Oral Pathology and Medicine. 2007;**36**(10):575-580

[11] Hsue SS, Wang WC, Chen CH, Lin CC, Chen YK, Lin LM. Malignant transformation in 1458 patients with potentially malignant oral mucosal disorders: A follow-up study based in a Taiwanese hospital. Journal of Oral Pathology and Medicine. 2007;**36**(1):25-29

[12] Bray F, Ferlay J, Laversanne M, Brewster DH, Gombe Mbalawa C, Kohler B, et al. Cancer incidence in five continents: Inclusion criteria, highlights from volume X and the global status of cancer registration. International Journal of Cancer. 2015;**137**(9):2060-2071

[13] Lambert R, Sauvaget C, Camargo CM, De, Sankaranarayanan R. Epidemiology of cancer from the oral cavity and oropharynx. European Journal of Gastroenterology and Hepatology. 2011;**23**(8):633-641

[14] Bhurgri Y, Bhurgri A, Usman A, Pervez S, Kayani N, et al. Epidemiological review of head and neck cancers in Karachi. Asian Pacific Journal of Cancer Prevention. 2006;**7**(2):195-200

[15] Tseng CH. Oral cancer in Taiwan: Is diabetes a risk factor? Clinical Oral Investigations. 2013;**17**(5):1357-1364

[16] Brown LM, Check DP, Devesa SS. Oropharyngeal cancer incidence trends: Diminishing racial disparities. Cancer Causes and Control. 2011;**22**(5):753-763

[17] Saba NF, Goodman M, Ward K, Flowers C, Ramalingam S, et al. Gender and ethnic disparities in incidence and survival of squamous cell carcinoma of the oral tongue, base of tongue, and tonsils: A surveillance, epidemiology and end results program-based analysis. Oncology. 2011;**81**(1):12-20

[18] Bonifazi M, Malvezzi M, Bertuccio P, Edefonti V, Garavello W, et al. Age-period-cohort analysis of oral cancer mortality in Europe: The end of an epidemic? Oral Oncology. 2011;**47**(5):400-407

[19] Yako-Suketomo H, Matsuda T. Comparison of time trends in lip, oral cavity and pharynx cancer mortality (1990-2006) between countries based on the WHO Mortality Database. Japanese Journal of Clinical Oncology. 2010;**40**(11):1118-1119

[20] Lim SS, Vos T, Flaxman AD, Danaei G, Shibuya K, Adair-Rohani H, et al. A comparative risk assessment of burden of disease and injury attributable to 67 risk factors and risk factor clusters in 21 regions, 1990-2010: A systematic analysis for the global burden of disease study 2010. The Lancet. 2012;**380**(9859):2224-2260

[21] World Cancer Research Fund, American Institute for Cancer Research. Food, Nutrition, Physical Activity, and the Prevention of Cancer: A Global Perspective. Washington: American Institute for Cancer Research; 2007

[22] Brown IJ, Tzoulaki I, Candeias V, Elliott P. Salt intakes around the world: Implications for public health. International Journal of Epidemiology. 2009;**38**(3):791-813

[23] Parkin DM. The evolution of the population-based cancer registry. Nature Reviews Cancer. 2006;**6**(8):603

[24] Center MM, Jemal A, Smith RA, Ward E. Worldwide variations in colorectal cancer. CA: A Cancer Journal for Clinicians. 2009;**59**(6):366-378

[25] Center MM, Jemal A, Ward E. International trends in colorectal cancer incidence rates. Cancer Epidemiology, Biomarkers and Prevention. 2009;**18**(6):1688-1694

[26] Bergstrom A, Pisani P, Tenet V, Wolk A, Adami HO. Overweight as an avoidable cause of cancer in Europe. International Journal of Cancer. 2001;**91**(3):421-430

[27] Renehan AG, Soerjomataram I, Tyson M, Egger M, Zwahlen M, Coebergh JW, et al. Incident cancer burden attributable to excess body mass index in 30 European countries. International Journal of Cancer. 2010;**126**(3):692-702

[28] Stevens GA, Singh GM, Lu Y, Danaei G, Lin JK, Finucane MM, et al. National, regional, and global trends in adult overweight and obesity prevalences. Population Health Metrics. 2012;**10**(1):22

[29] Lin D, Bucci MK, Eisele DW, Wang SJ. Squamous cell carcinoma of the buccal mucosa: A retrospective analysis of 22 cases. Ear, Nose, & Throat Journal. 2008;**87**:582-586

[30] Misra S, Chaturvedi A, Misra NC. Management of gingivobuccal complex cancer. Annals of the Royal College of Surgeons of England. 2008;**90**:546-553

[31] Nandakumar A. National cancer registry programme. Indian Council of Medical Research, Consolidated Report of the Population Based Cancer Registries, New Delhi, India; 1990. p. 96

[32] Rath GK, Parikh PM, Hukku S, Rajan B, Kumar S, Malhotra H, et al. Indian Council of Medical Research consensus document for the management of buccal mucosa cancer. Indian Journal of Medical and Paediatric Oncology: Official Journal of Indian Society of Medical & Paediatric Oncology. 2014;**35**(2):136

[33] Kato H, Kanematsu M, Watanabe H, Mizuta K, Aoki M. Metastatic retropharyngeal lymph nodes: Comparison of CT and MR imaging for diagnostic accuracy. European Journal of Radiology. 2014;**83**(7):1157-1162

[34] Liu LZ, Zhang GY, Xie CM, Liu XW, Cui CY, Li L. Magnetic resonance imaging of retropharyngeal lymph node metastasis in nasopharyngeal carcinoma: Patterns of spread. International Journal of Radiation Oncology, Biology, Physics. 2006;**66**(3):721-730

[35] Reis PP, Waldron L, Perez-Ordonez B, Pintilie M, Galloni NN, Xuan Y, et al. A gene signature in histologically normal surgical margins is predictive of oral carcinoma recurrence. BMC Cancer. 2011;**11**(1):437

[36] O'donnell RK, Kupferman M, Wei SJ, Singhal S, Weber R, O'Malley B Jr, et al. Gene expression signature predicts lymphatic metastasis in squamous cell carcinoma of the oral cavity. Oncogene. 2005;**24**(7):1244

[37] Coelho KR. Challenges of the oral cancer burden in India. Journal of Cancer Epidemiology. 2012;**2012**:1-17

[38] Hamoir M, Schmitz S, Suarez C, Strojan P, Hutcheson K, Rodrigo J, et al. The current role of salvage surgery in recurrent head and neck squamous cell carcinoma. Cancers. 2018;**10**(8):267

[39] Estilo CL, Pornchai O, Talbot S, Socci ND, Carlson DL, Ghossein R, et al. Oral tongue cancer gene expression profiling: Identification of novel potential prognosticators by oligonucleotide microarray analysis. BMC Cancer. 2009;**9**(1):11

[40] Jerjes W, Upile T, Petrie A, Riskalla A, Hamdoon Z, Vourvachis M, et al. Clinicopathological parameters, recurrence, locoregional and distant metastasis in 115 T1-T2 oral squamous cell carcinoma patients. Head & Neck Oncology. 2010;**2**(1):9

[41] Diaz EM, Holsinger C, Zuniga E. Squamous cell carcinoma of the buccal mucosa: One institution's experience with 119 previously untreated patients. Head and Neck. 2003;**25**(4):267-273

[42] Shaw RJ, McGlashan G, Worlgar JA, Zowe D, Brown JS, Vanghan ED, et al. Prognostic importance of site in squamous cell carcinoma of buccal mucosa. British Journal of Oral and Maxillofacial Surgery. 2009;**47**:356-359

[43] Van't Veer LJ, Dai H, van de Vijver MJ, He YD, Hart AA, Mao M, et al. Gene expression profiling predicts clinical outcome of breast cancer. Nature. 2002;**415**:530-536

[44] Ramaswamy S, Ross KN, Lander ES, Golub TR. A molecular signature of metastasis in primary solid tumors. Nature Genetics. 2002;**33**(1):49

[45] Nathan CA, Amirghahri N, Rice C, Abreo FW, Shi R, Stucker FJ. Molecular analysis of surgical margins in head and neck squamous cell carcinoma patients. The Laryngoscope. 2002;**112**(12):2129-2140

[46] Bilde A, von Buchwald C, Dabelsteen E, Therkildsen MH, Dabelsteen S. Molecular markers in the surgical margin of oral carcinomas. Journal of Oral Pathology & Medicine. 2009;**38**(1):72-78

[47] Tan HK, Saulnier P, Auperin A, Lacroix L, Casiraghi O, Janot F, et al. Quantitative methylation analyses of resection margins predict local recurrences and disease-specific deaths in patients with head and neck squamous cell carcinomas. British Journal of Cancer. 2008;**99**(2):357-363

[48] Nathan CA, Franklin S, Abreo FW, Nassar R, De Benedetti A, Glass J. Analysis of surgical margins with the molecular marker eIF4E: A prognostic factor in patients with head and neck cancer. Journal of Clinical Oncology. 1999;**17**(9):2909-2914

[49] Van der Toorn PP, Veltman JA, Bot FJ, de Jong JM, Manni JJ, Ramaekers FC, et al. Mapping of resection margins of oral cancer for p53 overexpression and chromosome instability to detect residual (pre)malignant cells. The Journal of Pathology. 2001;**193**(1):66-72

[50] Cox S, Vickers ER, Ghu S, Zoellner H. Salivary arecoline levels during areca nut chewing in human volunteers. Journal of Oral Pathology and Medicine. 2010;**39**(6):465-469

[51] Sharan RN, Mehrotra R, Choudhury Y, Asotra K. Association of betel nut with carcinogenesis: Revisit with a clinical perspective. PLoS One. 2012;**7**(8):e42759

[52] Shieh DH, Chiang LC, Lee CH, Yang YH, Shieh TY. Effects of arecoline, safrole, and nicotine on collagen phagocytosis by human buccal mucosal fibroblasts as a possible mechanism for oral submucous fibrosis in Taiwan. Journal of Oral Pathology and Medicine. 2004;**33**(9):581-587

[53] Pindborg JJ, Reibel J, Holmstrup P. Subjectivity in evaluating oral epithelial dysplasia, carcinoma in situ and initial carcinoma. Journal of Oral Pathology. 1985;**14**:698-708

[54] Abbey LM, Kaugars GE, Gunsolley JC, Burns JC, Page DG, Svirsky JA, et al. Intra examiner and inter examiner reliability in the diagnosis of oral epithelial dysplasia. Oral Surgery, Oral Medicine, Oral Pathology, Oral Radiology, and Endodontology. 1995;**80**:188-191

[55] Karabulut A, Reibel J, Therkildsen MH, Praetorius F, Nielsen HW, Dabelsteen E. Observer variability in the histologic assessment of oral premalignant lesions. Journal of Oral Pathology & Medicine. 1995;**24**:198-200

[56] Sudbø J, Bryne M, Johannessen AC, Kildal W, Danielsen HE, Reith A. Comparison of histological grading and large-scale genomic status (DNA ploidy) as prognostic tools in oral dysplasia. The Journal of Pathology. 2001;**194**:303-310

[57] Patel PN, Mehta M, Goyal S, Gohil M, Suryanarayana U. Results of 2 dimensional post-operative radiotherapy treatment in carcinoma buccal mucosa patients: A regional cancer centre experience. Acta Medica International. 2016;**3**(2):116

[58] Diaz EM, Holsinger FC, Zuniga ER, Roberts DB, Sorensen DM. Squamous cell carcinoma of the buccal mucosa: One institution's experience with 119 previously untreated patients. Head and Neck. 2003;**25**:267-273

[59] Mishra RC, Parida TK, Mohanty S. Tumour thickness and relationship to locoregional failure in cancer of the buccal mucosa. European Journal of Surgical Oncology. 1999;**25**:186-189

[60] Borges AM, Shrikhande SS, Ganesh B. Surgical pathology of squamous carcinoma of the oral cavity: Its impact in management. Seminars in Surgical Oncology. 1989;**5**:310-317

[61] Alizadeh AA, Eisen MB, Davis RE, Ma C, Lossos IS, Rosenwald A, et al. Distinct types of diffuse large B-cell lymphoma identified by gene expression profiling. Nature. 2000;**403**(6769):503

[62] Beer DG, Kardia SL, Huang CC, Giordano TJ, Levin AM, Misek DE, et al. Gene-expression profiles predict survival of patients with lung adenocarcinoma. Nature Medicine. 2002;**8**(8):816

[63] Jones AS, Hanafi ZB, Nadapalan V, Roland NJ, Kinsella A, Helliwell TR. Do positive resection margins after ablative surgery for head and neck cancer adversely affect prognosis? A study of 352 patients with recurrent carcinoma following radiotherapy treated by salvage surgery. British Journal of Cancer. 1996;**74**(1):128

[64] Leemans CR, Tiwari R, Nauta JJ, Waal IV, Snow GB. Recurrence at the primary site in head and neck cancer and the significance of neck lymph node metastases as a prognostic factor. Cancer. 1994;**73**(1):187-190

[65] Sticht C, Freier K, Knopfle K, Flechtenmacher C, Pungs S, Hofele C, et al. Activation of MAP kinase signaling through ERK5 but not ERK1 expression is associated with lymph node metastases in oral squamous cell carcinoma (OSCC). Neoplasia. 2008;**10**(5):462-470

[66] Dabelsteen E, Clausen H, Mandel U. Aberrant glycosylation in oral malignant and premalignant lesions. Journal of Oral Pathology and Medicine. 1991;**20**(8):361-368

[67] Paterson IC, Eveson JW, Prime SS. Molecular changes in oral cancer may reflect aetiology and ethnic origin. European Journal of Cancer Part B. Oral Oncology. 1996;**32**(3):150-153

[68] Cardoso F. Microarray technology and its effect on breast cancer (re) classification and prediction of outcome. Breast Cancer Research. 2003;**5**(6):303

[69] Drukker CA, Bueno-de-Mesquita JM, Retèl VP, van Harten WH, van Tinteren H, Wesseling J, et al. A prospective evaluation of a breast cancer prognosis signature in the observational RASTER study. International Journal of Cancer. 2013;**133**(4):929-936

[70] Hainsworth JD, Greco FA. Treatment of patients with cancer of an unknown primary site. The New England Journal of Medicine. 1993;**329**(4):257-263

[71] Bièche I, Tozlu S, Girault I, Lidereau R. Identification of a three-gene expression signature of poor-prognosis breast carcinoma. Molecular Cancer. 2004;**3**(1):37

[72] Abendstein H, Nordgren M, Boysen M, Jannert M, Silander E, Ahlner-Elmqvist M, et al. Quality of life and head and neck cancer: A 5 year prospective study. The Laryngoscope. 2005;**115**(12):2183-2192

[73] Sherman AC, Simonton S, Adams DC, Vural E, Owens B, Hanna E. Assessing quality of life in patients with head and neck cancer: Cross-validation of the European Organization for Research and Treatment of Cancer (EORTC) quality of life head and neck module (QLQ-H&N35). Archives of Otolaryngology - Head and Neck Surgery. 2000;**126**(4):459-467

[74] Cognetti DM, Weber RS, Lai SY. Head and neck cancer: An evolving treatment paradigm. Cancer. 2008;**113**(S7):1911-1932

Chapter 2

Laser Dental Treatment Techniques

Zahra Jassim Mohammed Al Timimi and
Mohammed Saleem Ismail Alhabeel

Additional information is available at the end of the chapter

http://dx.doi.org/10.5772/intechopen.80029

Abstract

Dental laser technologies are one of the most rapidly developing areas in the modern technology. When the laser was discovered in the 1960s, it was classified as a solution in search of a problem, and today, laser technology is applied in many different areas. It basically remained a field of research. Typically in the most frequent dental surgery, the caries therapy was frequently compared to most types of lasers; the conventional mechanical drills are still superior, particularly CW or long-pulse lasers. Only laser systems capable of providing ultrashort pulses might be an alternative to mechanical drills. The number of laser applications is enormous, and it is not possible to explain all of them here. In this chapter, the development of suitable application units for laser radiation and other topics of interest in dentistry including laser treatment of soft tissue as well as laser welding of dental bridges and dentures are discussed. In some of these areas, research has been very successful. However, many clinical studies and extensive engineering effort still remain to be done in order to achieve satisfactory results.

Keywords: dental laser, dentistry, tissue interaction, radiation, wavelength

1. Introduction

1.1. Review of laser physics and tissue interaction

LASER is an acronym for light amplification by stimulated emission of radiation, which is based on theories and principles first put forth by Einstein in the early 1900s [1]. Laser light has a single wavelength. The production of lasing occurs when an excited atom is stimulated to release a photon before it occurs spontaneously. The spontaneous emission results in random light waves alike to light emitted by a light bulb [2]. The stimulated emission of photons produces a very coherent, collimated, and monochromatic radiation that is found nowhere else in nature [3]. Because laser radiation is so concentrated and focused, it may have an effect on target tissue at a much lower energy level than the other light sources [4]. The effects of laser radiation on the target tissue are dependent on its wavelength, power, and spot size

Laser type	Wavelengths	Delivery systems	Applications
CO_2	10,600 nm	Pulse or continuous wave	1. Soft tissue ablation 2. Gingival contouring for esthetic purposes 3. Treatment of oral ulcerative lesions 4. Frenectomy and gingivectomy 5. Elimination of necrotic epithelial tissue during regenerative periodontal surgeries
Nd:YAG	1064 nm	Pulse	6. Root canal therapy: helps eliminate pathogenic microorganisms and debris from the root canal 7. Extensive periodontal surgery and scaling to eliminate necrotic tissues and pathogenic microorganisms 8. Caries removal
Er:YAG	2940 nm	Pulse	9. Caries removal 10. Cavity preparation in enamel and dentin 11. Root canal preparation
Er,Cr:YSGG	2780 nm	Pulse	12. Enamel etching 13. Caries removal 14. Cavity preparation 15. Bone ablation without overheating, melting, or changing the calcium and phosphorus ratios 16. Root canal preparation
Argon	572 nm	Pulse or continuous wave	17. Polymerization of restorative resin materials 18. Tooth bleaching 19. Elimination of necrotic tissue and gingival contouring 20. Treatment of oral lesions such as recurrent aphthous ulcers or herpetic lesions 21. Frenectomy and gingivectomy
Diode	810–980 nm	Pulse or continuous wave	22. Proliferation of fibroblasts and enhancing the healing of oral lesions or surgical wounds 23. Frenectomy and gingivectomy 24. Correcting the gingival contouring for esthetic purposes
HO:YAG	2100 nm	Pulse	25. Gingival contouring 26. Treatment of oral lesions 27. Frenectomy and gingivectomy

Table 1. Lasers types, wavelengths, and their dental applications.

which is determined by the laser device [5]. If the laser radiation comes into contact with the tissue, it can reflect, scatter, absorbed, or be transmitted to the other surrounding tissues. In the biological tissue, the absorption of laser radiation occurs because of the presence of free water molecules, proteins, pigments, and even other organic matters [6, 7]. Thermal interactions caused by the laser radiation, the water molecules, and their absorption coefficient perform a strong role [1]. Laser beams (*Er,Cr:YSGG, Er:YAG*) are well absorbed by water which are able to mechanically ablate enamel, dentin, and alveolar bone, while laser beams (*diode, Nd:YAG,* CO_2) are not well absorbed by water, resulting in strong thermal reactions, such as carbonization, charring, and melting of organic tissue [8, 9].

1.2. Review of modern laser technology accessible in dentistry

The first investigation of using the laser in dentistry was within the surrounding hard tissue, such as cavity preparation and caries removal as a replacement for the conventional drill. The ruby laser that was the focus of this investigation was invented in 1960 [10]. In succeeding years, many researchers examined the hard-tissue applications of the laser by using different types of lasers such as Ar, CO_2, and Nd:YAG. However, some studies resulted in major thermal damage to enamel and dentin [11], while other researchers concentrated their attention on the laser applications on soft tissue of these early generation high-powered lasers. It was determined that the CO_2 and the Nd:YAG lasers were capable of excellent soft tissue ablation and hemostasis [12]. These studies enabled the periodontists to use these lasers for soft-tissue treatment, such as gingivectomies and frenectomies [13, 14]. Despite, these early studies profound a thermal effect on target tissues, including gingiva, periodontal ligament, cementum, and alveolar bone, that their using for periodontal hard tissue was not promising. Within the 1990s, the Nd:YAG laser was included that had a flexible and fiber-optic delivery system, which made it appropriate for periodontal pocket, including the root surface debridement and pocket curettage [15, 16].

Researchers concluded that the Er:YAG laser, which is highly absorbed by water and hydroxyapatite, had an effect in enamel cutting [17, 18]. Subsequently, Eversole and others published numerous distinguished researches on the Er,Cr:YSGG laser and its effectiveness in soft tissue application (enamel, dentin, and bone), which all play a significant performance in periodontal [19, 20].

Because of this versatility, the Er,Cr:YSGG laser was the first all-in-one laser that made an economics of providing a laser treatment and more feasible for the periodontist and general practitioner [21]. Over the time, the collective research has resulted in a laser that has a real and beneficial application for periodontal care. Laser types, wavelengths, and their applications are listed in **Table 1**.

2. Dental laser systems and the basics of the work

2.1. Basic processes of laser radiation and tissue interaction

One of the main difficulties of all starting dental laser using is the depth of penetration of laser to the tissue and its effects on the principal constituents of the tissue. In order to clarify these questions, it is necessary to consider the process of light penetration in the tissue and the biological effects on the tissue [9, 22].

The process of laser penetration in the biological tissues is extremely complicated. This was connected to others with their nonhomogeneous structure. From the dental point of view, it is very necessary to deliver precisely a respective dosage of laser energy to a given tissue [2, 20].

This energy will be absorbed and transformed into other forms of energy. The laser passing through the upper layers of the tissue is reflected, scattered, and partially absorbed [23]. A degree of these processes is dependent upon tissue type and in the case of the epidermis. It can differ from the case of the skin or oil gland irradiation. In order to define the tissue laser radiation interaction, some considerations should be addressed with respect to the physical parameters and the structural features of the irradiated tissue [10, 12]. The absorption limit and its width are conditional upon the tissue structure, water, hemoglobin, enamel, dentin, pulp cavity, etc. [24].

Anyhow, the process of laser tissue radiation interaction is determined by the wavelength, power, and the irradiation time. The primary characteristics of this interaction are illustrated in **Figures 1** and **2**. **Figure 1** shows the primary physical phenomena, transmission, reflection, scattering, and absorption which occur including the biological tissue.

If there are two materials, one is white and the second black, in the sunlight, the white body will reflect more light waves than the black one and it will be cooler than the black body, which absorbs more solar energy. The radiation of the tissue involves the release of these four processes simultaneously [11, 25].

The transmission and the absorption of the laser in the given tissue are dependent, apart from its wavelength, and upon its power, it is not dependent on irradiation time. The spot size of the laser beam and its intensity will be the same regardless of how long this laser is on [26].

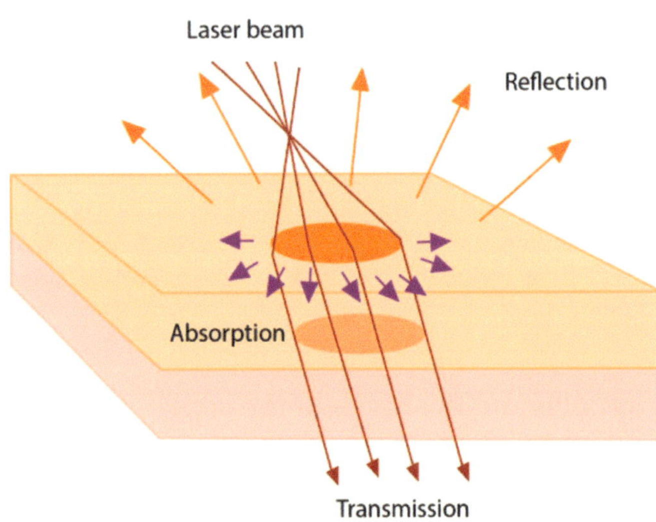

Figure 1. Illustration of the basic phenomena always accompanying the light-tissue interaction [28].

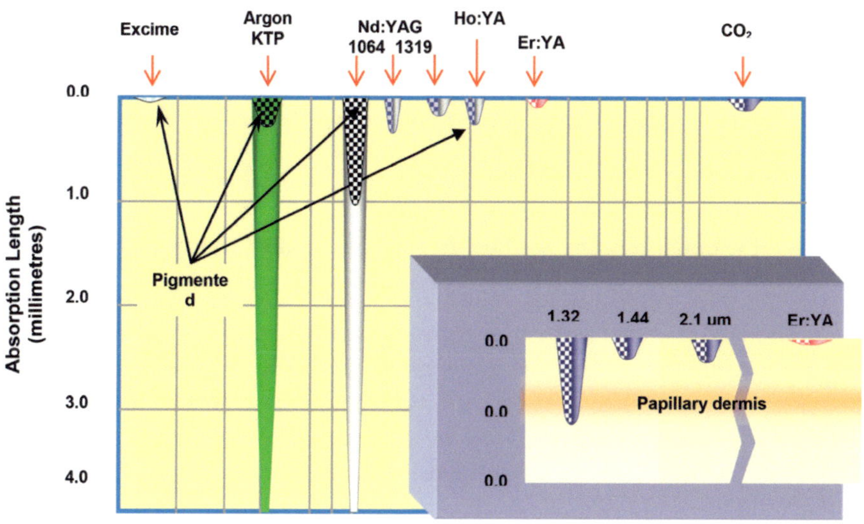

Figure 2. Transmission values of the main wavelengths for selected parts of the skin.

For example, the laser source with an output power of 30 mW emits 10^{16} photons per second. Theoretically, that means 10^{16} photons penetrate in the tissue every second [15]. Accordingly, it does not matter if a given point is irradiated for 1 second or for 1 minute. The alike situation occurs when we shine a given point on the wall with an electric torch [1, 5, 27].

The point is to select the wavelengths in bands where the processes of effective transmission in tissues for biostimulation purposes are predominant as well as for cutting, coagulation, defects, etc.

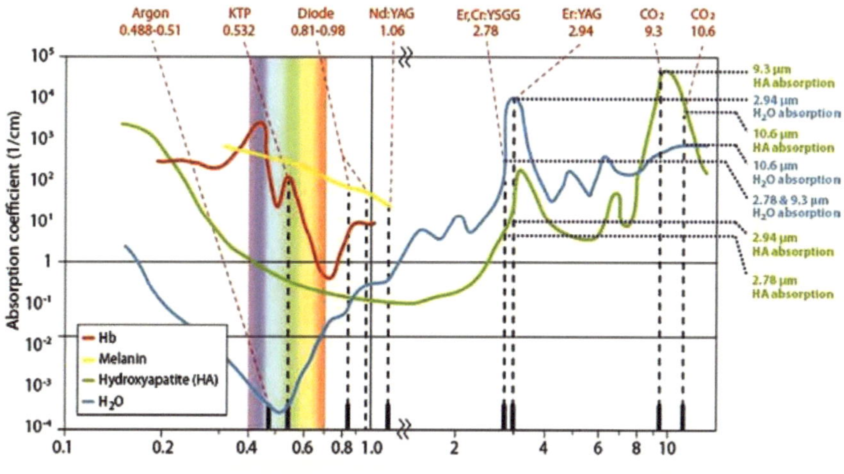

Figure 3. Characteristic of absorption of the laser light for the main tissue components [13].

Figure 2 shows in detail the transmission of the major important laser wavelengths in particular constituents of the skin tissue, while **Figure 3** illustrates the optical absorption characteristics of water, hemoglobin, and melanin and shows precisely the primary constituents of the tissue where absorption covers 100%.

Figure 4 displays the curves of the absorption by the principal components of teeth tissues and laser wavelengths. The biggest absorption occurs with wavelength of approximately 2900 nm. This is the radiation generated by Er:YAG laser and CO_2 laser radiation—10,600 nm ranks second, respectively. The abovementioned dependence for particular tooth tissues.

The time duration of treatment session on a given point is significant since it determined the total number of the photons penetrated in the tissue [25]. Photons emitted by laser source do not penetrate into deeper tissue layers even if a given point is irradiated for a longer time [5, 29]. If we mention the above example with the electric torch, we can see that the laser beam will not reach further and it is not more intensive, no matter whether the laser is on for an hour or for a minute.

In spite of this explanation, the treatment effect is obtained in a deeper layer after the long period of laser irradiation. This phenomenon occurring is similar to the exponential dependence between the transmitted energy (total number of photons transmitted during a therapeutic session) and the depth of penetration [3, 29].

The relation between the time duration of a treatment session and therapeutic effects can be explained by the penetrating photons that initiate the chain reaction which transfers the biological effects of the therapeutic session to the deeper tissue layers and at sides [30].

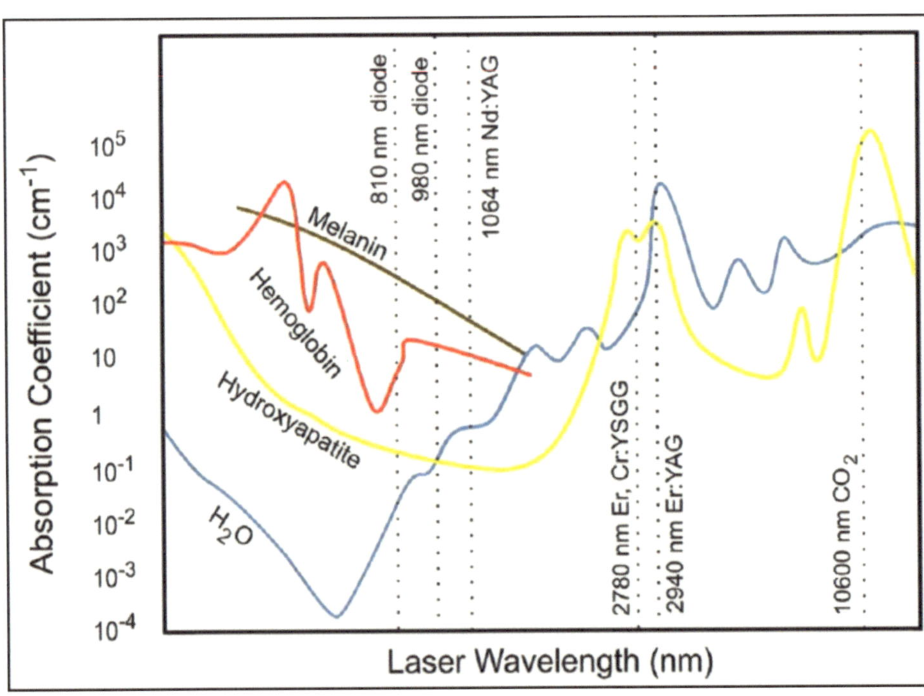

Figure 4. Characteristics of laser beam absorption as the function of wavelength for the main components of the tooth [26].

http://dx.doi.org/10.5772/intechopen.80029

3. Clinical applications and descriptions

3.1. Laser treatment of hard tooth substance (enamel and dentin)

The carious material contains a higher content of water compared with other surrounding dental healthy hard tissues. As a result, the ablation efficiency of caries is higher than other healthy tissues. There was a possible selectivity in removing carious material by using Er:YAG laser because of the various energy dose requirements to ablate the carious and also healthy tissue leaving those healthy tissues minimally affected. It was found that the Er:YAG laser can ablate the carious dentin effectively with the minimal thermal damage to the other surrounding intact dentins [19, 31, 32] (**Figures 5–8**).

The laser can remove infected and softened carious dentin to the same degree as the bur treatment [33]. However, the lower degree of vibration was remarked with the Er:YAG laser treatment (see **Figures 10–14**).

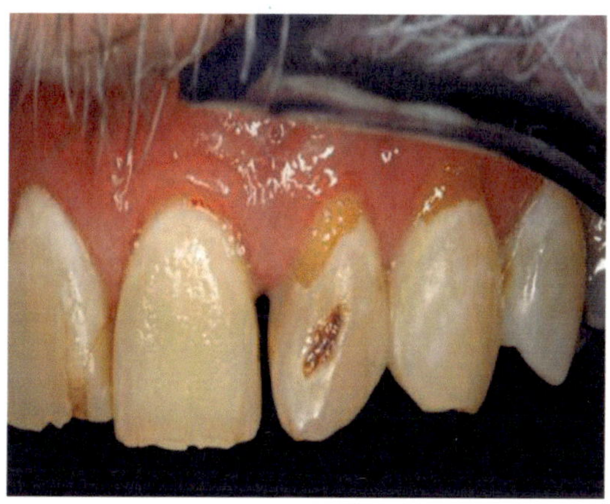

Figure 5. Decay present on the facial of the maxillary left lateral incisor.

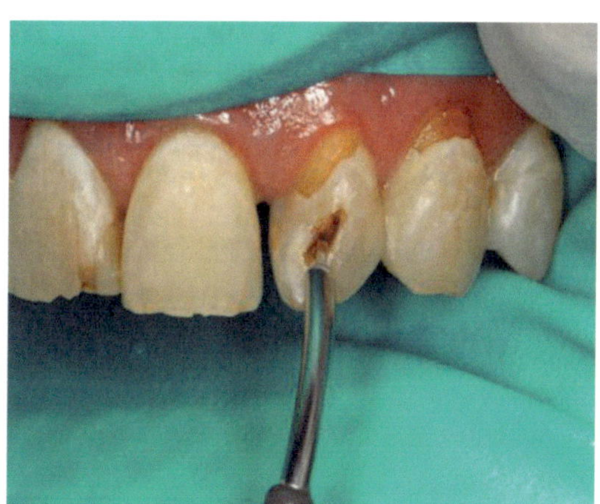

Figure 6. The erbium laser used to remove the decay. No anesthesia was required.

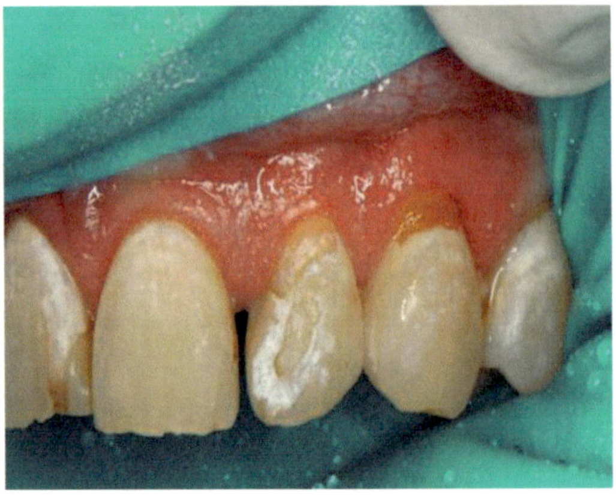

Figure 7. After caries removal and preparation is complete.

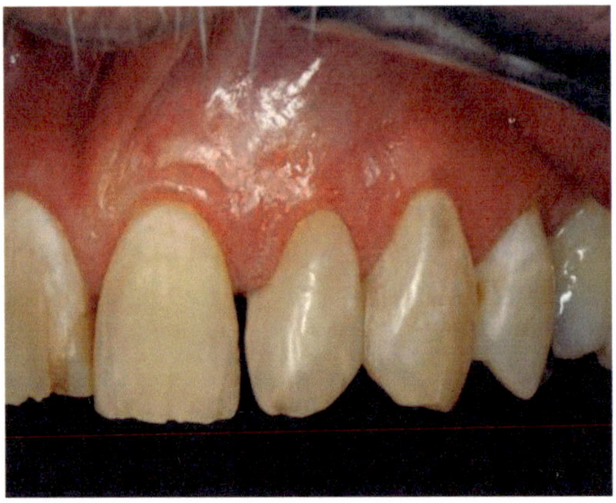

Figure 8. Definitive direct-bonded restoration after preparation with the erbium laser [33].

The YSGG laser was cleared for classes I, II, III, IV, and V cavity preps, as well as caries removal, in 1999, with a similar clearance for children soon thereafter (1999). Since then, published reports have demonstrated the laser's ability to reduce and even eliminate the smear layer associated with traditional rotary instruments which can improve surface adhesion and bond strength for restorations [18, 20].

Also, because the laser reacts at a cellular level and helps to prohibit the pain response, most hard-tissue procedures can be completed without the aid of injected anesthetic [10].

The YSGG laser provides the precise treatment of pits and fissures on the occlusal surfaces of the molars as shown in **Figures 9** and **10**, which has aided in the growing discipline of "micro" and "minimally invasive" dentistry.

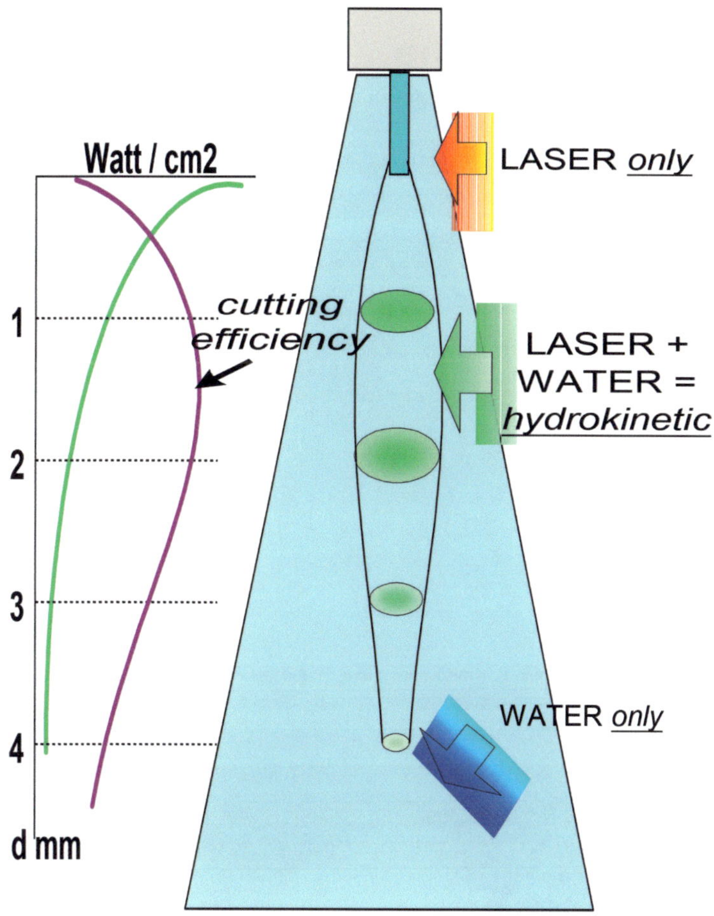

Figure 9. Cutting with YSGG (Waterlase). Optimization of the cutting efficiency: distance to tissue should be maintained at 1–2 mm (when power and spray are at proper settings).

3.2. Soft tissue

3.2.1. Periodontal disease

The YSGG laser was the exclusive laser evacuated for major indications in periodontal therapy, while other lasers such as the diode laser or Nd:YAG are absolved for soft tissue applications related to perio; none have been cleared for cutting oral osseous tissues, a core component of any periodontal program [34]. See **Figures 11–13**.

The YSGG laser was approved by the FDA for a wide array of indications related to the periodontal health like laser curettage, sulcular debridement, ostectomy, soft tissue flap elevation, removing of pathological tissues from bony sockets, and other related clinical applications [35].

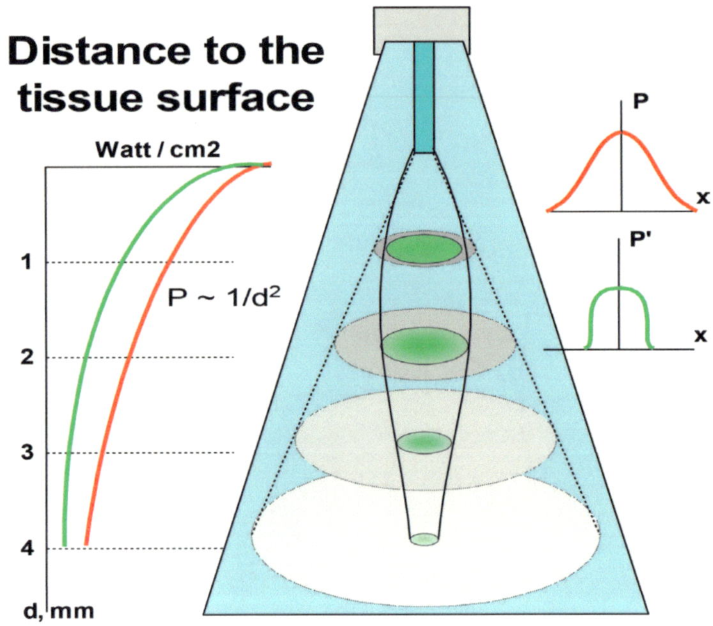

Figure 10. YSGG (Waterlase) parameters. Radiation wavelength and power (energy) density. To reduce cutting speed with Waterlase—"defocus," back off from tissue; there is optimal distance range to cut tissue.

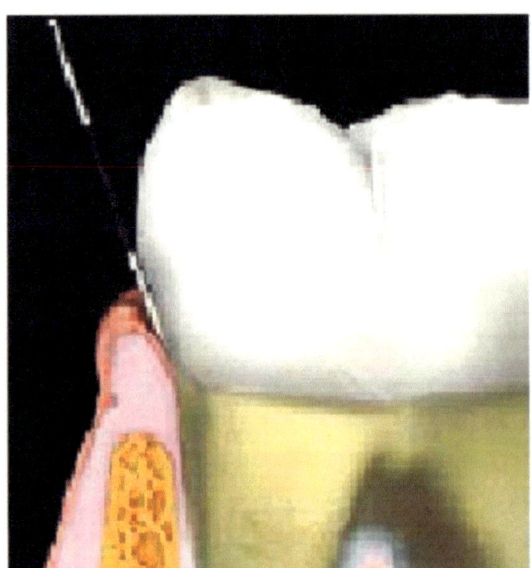

Figure 11. Hand scaling [35].

3.2.2. *Removal of oral pyogenic granuloma*

A variety of benign soft tissue swellings can be found arising from oral mucosa, most of which are inflammatory hyperplasia and granuloma. These lesions can be divided into those which

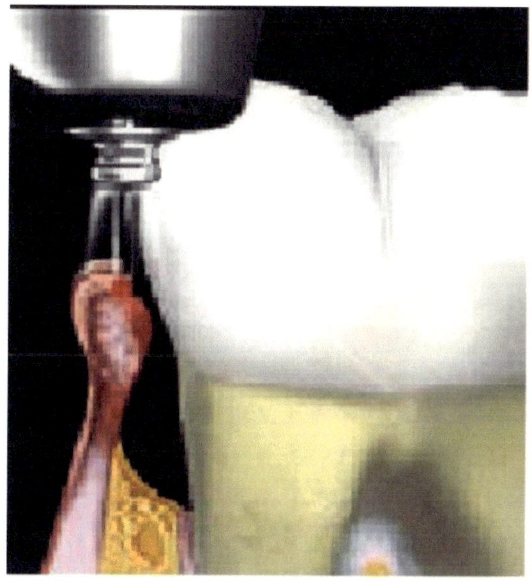

Figure 12. Laser-assisted scaling using the Er,Cr:YSGG laser [35].

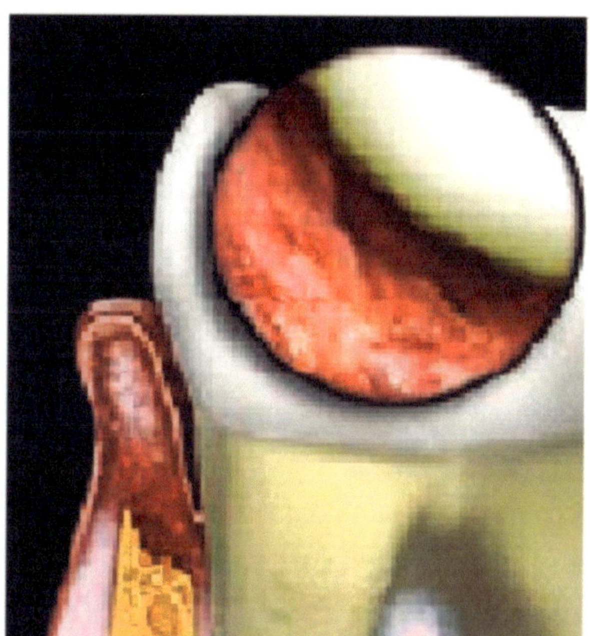

Figure 13. Thoroughly debrided root surface [35].

arise from the mucosa covering the alveolar processes and those which arise elsewhere in the oral cavity [36]. The soft tissue masses which are excised should be sent for histological examination.

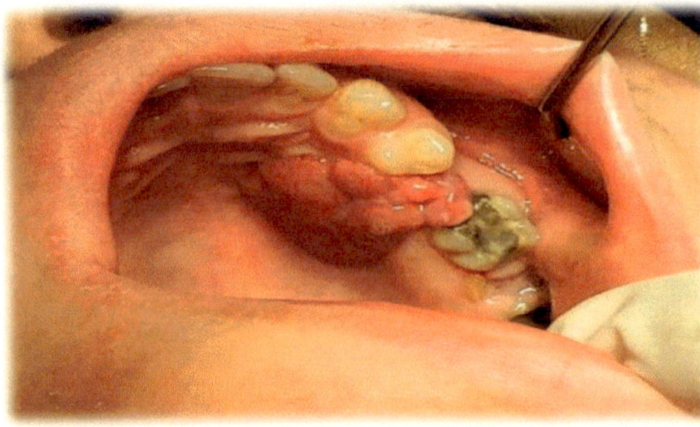

Figure 14. Pyogenic granuloma of the left side of palatal mucosa [8].

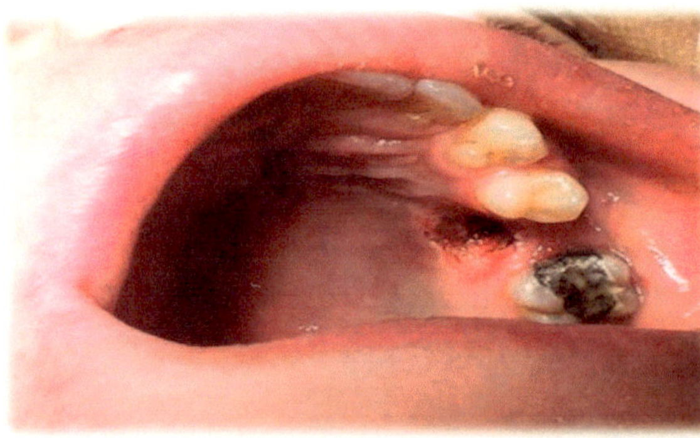

Figure 15. Complete excision of granuloma by diode laser 5 W pulsed mode [8].

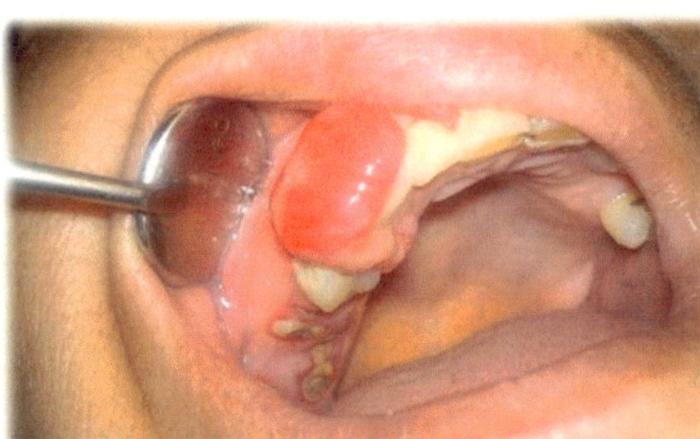

Figure 16. Pyogenic granuloma of the right side of maxillary alveolar mucosa [8].

A study by Mahmood et al. [8] has enrolled 35 patients with oral pyogenic granuloma. The type of laser, which was used in this study, is a diode laser with 810 nm wavelength, gallium aluminum arsenide (GaAlAs), output power of 15 W, and pulse duration between

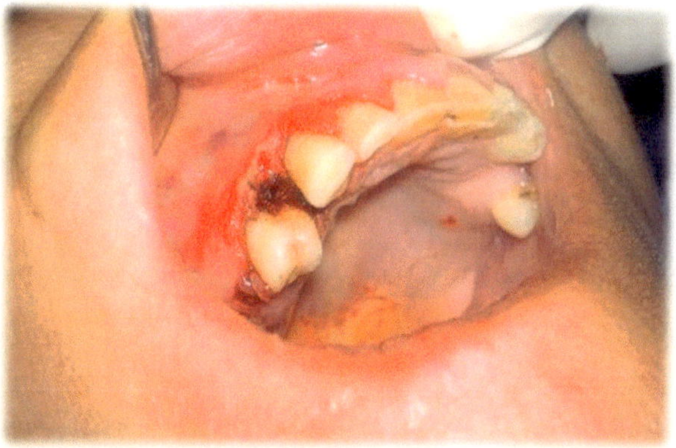

Figure 17. Complete excision of granuloma by diode laser 5 W pulsed mode [8].

0.1 and 1.0 second and works in continuous, single, and repeated pulsed modes. The laser surgical operations had been done at repetitive pulsed mode for 5–8 W maximum power, 0.2–0.4 seconds pulse duration, and 0.2–0.4 seconds pulse interval. The results were evaluated clinically depending on swelling, infection, disturbance of function, pain, and bleeding. The postoperative swelling was minimal to moderate. No sutures were required. No bleeding was seen neither intraoperative nor postoperative period. Postoperative pain was mild in few patients. No disturbance of function was observed [8] (**Figures 14–17**).

4. Conclusion

Using the laser dramatically can reduce the need of applying a high-speed drill to the tooth surface for any reason. Nevertheless, it was not yet to completely replace the drill because a laser cannot effectively cut reflective surfaces such as the metal and the porcelain.

The fact that a single instrument can remove the bulk amounts of enamel, dentin, and decay and then cut the soft tissue around the area typically requires an anesthetic to take the effect. It observes an exciting new era of effective laser dentistry.

The YSGG laser has practical viable applications across a wide clinical spectrum like hard tissue, soft tissue, bone, endo, and perio, and because it has utility in both hard and soft tissue applications, the Er,Cr:YSGG laser outperforms other conventional modalities in many ways.

Conflict of interest

The author declares no conflict of interest, financial or otherwise.

Author details

Zahra Jassim Mohammed Al Timimi[1]* and Mohammed Saleem Ismail Alhabeel[2]

*Address all correspondence to: dr.altimimizahra@gmail.com, zahraja2007@yahoo.com and dentosemo@yahoo.com

1 Laser Physics-College of Science for Women, Babylon University, Iraq

2 ABLS, Development for Laser Dentistry, Middle East and Europe

References

[1] Zahra A-T. Exploration of additional mechanical phenomena of laser-tissue interaction contributes to the damage and elimination of the small blood vessels. The International Journal of Scientific & Engineering Research [Internet]. 2014;**5**:672-675. Available from: https://www.ijser.org/onlineResearchPaperViewer.aspx?Exploration-of-Additional-Mechanical-Phenomena-of-Laser-Tissue.pdf

[2] Al Timimi Z, Jaafar M, Zubir Mat Jafri M. Photodynamic therapy and green laser blood therapy. Global Journal of Medicine Research [Internet]. 2011;**11**:22-28. Available from: http://www.isla-laser.org/wp-content/uploads/5-Photodynamic-therapy-and-Green-Laser-blood-Therapy.pdf

[3] Hamad F, Jaafar M, Hamid A, et al. Influences of different low level laser power at wavelength 635 nm for two types of skin; dark and light. Proceedings of the 7th IMT-GT UNINET and the 3rd International PSU-UNS Conference on Bioscience. 2009;**7**:130-135

[4] Zahra A-T, Mustafa FH, HAA H. Characterization of cancer photodynamic therapy: Exploring the effects of hematoporphyrin derivative photosensitizer and low intensity laser irradiation. International Journal of Current Microbiology and Applied Sciences [Internet]. 2017;**6**:1-8. Available from: https://doi.org/10.20546/ijcmas

[5] Suhaimi MJ, Zahra JAT. Therapeutic laser for chronic low back pain. Bangladesh Journal of Medical Sciences [Internet]. October 2009;**4**:118-128. Available from: https://doi.org/10.3329/bjms.v8i4.4709

[6] Al Timimi Z, Jaafar MS, Jafri MZM, Houssein HAA, Mustafa FH. The influence of low power laser energy on red blood cell and platelets in vitro. International Conference on Bioscience, Biochemistry and Pharmaceutical Sciences (ICBBPS'2012) Penang, Malaysia. [Internet]. Penang, Malaysia; 2012. pp. 12-14. Available from: https://www.researchgate.net/publication/249970680_The_Influence_of_low-power_laser_Energy_on_Red_blood_cell_and_platelets_In_vitro

[7] Zahra A-T. Investigating the effects of green laser irradiation on red blood cells: green laser blood therapy. International Journal of Applied Research and Studies [Internet]. 2014;**3**:1-5. Available from: http://www.ijars.ijarsgroup.com/article.php?aToken=1543843a4723ed2ab08e18053ae6dc5b

[8] Mahmood S, Abolhab R, Mohamed M. The effectiveness of diode laser 810 nm in the removal of oral pyogenic granuloma in repetitive pulsed mode. The Iraqi Journal of Medical Sciences. 2015;**213**(2):137-142

[9] Adams TC, Pang PK. Lasers in aesthetic dentistry. Dental Clinics of North America. 2004:833-860

[10] Lakshmi MS, Goyal R. Lasers in paediatric dentistry. Journal of Evolution of Medical and Dental Sciences. 2014;**3**(51):11991-11998

[11] Van As G. Erbium lasers in dentistry. Dental Clinics of North America. 2004:1017-1059

[12] Goldman L, Goldman B, Van LN. Current laser dentistry. Lasers in Surgery and Medicine. 1987;**6**(6):559-562

[13] Dostálová T, Jelínková H. Lasers in dentistry. Lasers in Medical Application [Internet]. Elsevier. 2013:604-627. Available from: http://linkinghub.elsevier.com/retrieve/pii/B9780857092373500205

[14] Coluzzi DJ, Convissar RA. Lasers in clinical dentistry. Dental Clinics of North America. 2004;**48**(4)

[15] Featherstone JDB, Fried D. Fundamental interactions of lasers with dental hard tissues. Medical Laser Application. 2001:181-194

[16] White JM, Swift EJ. Lasers for use in dentistry. Journal of Esthetic and Restorative Dentistry [Internet]. 2005;**17**:60. Available from: http://dx.doi.org/10.1111/j.1708-8240.2005.tb00085.x

[17] Boari HGD, Ana PA, Eduardo CP, et al. Absorption and thermal study of dental enamel when irradiated with Nd:YAG laser with the aim of caries prevention. Laser Physics [Internet]. 2009;**19**(7):1463-1469. Available from: http://link.springer.com/10.1134/S1054660X09070160

[18] Walsh LJ. The current status of laser applications in dentistry. Australian Dental Journal. 2003;**48**(3):146-155

[19] Weiner GP. Laser dentistry practice management. Dental Clinics of North America. 2004:1105-1126

[20] Zahra A-T. Clinical evaluation of scalpel Er: YAG laser 2940 nm and conventional surgery incisions wound after oral soft tissue biopsy. Bangladesh Medical Research Council Bulletin [Internet]. 2018;**43**(3):149. Available from: https://www.banglajol.info/index.php/BMRCB/article/view/36429/24567

[21] Karu T. Laser biostimulation: A photobiological phenomenon. Journal of Photochemistry and Photobiology B: Biology. 1989:638

[22] Zahra'a A-T. Assessment of the impacts of 830 nm low power laser on triiodothyronine (T3), thyroxine (T4) and the thyroid stimulating hormone (TSH) in the rabbits. Journal of Medical Science and Clinical Research [Internet]. 2014;**2**:2902-2910. Available from: http://jmscr.igmpublication.org/home/index.php/archive/133-volume-02-issue-11-november-2014-in-process#13-2-abstract

[23] Welch AJ, Torres JH, Wai FC. Laser physics and laser tissue interaction. Laser Physics [Internet]. 1989;**61**:961-964. Available from: http://www.ncbi.nlm.nih.gov/pubmed/20118342

[24] Penetrante BM, Bardsley JN. Residual energy in plasmas produced by intense subpicosecond lasers. Physical Review A. 1991;**43**:3100-3113

[25] Zahra A, Timimi MS, Jaafar MZMJ. Comparison between low level laser therapy and exercise for treatment of chronic low back pain. Indian Journal of Physiotherapy & Occ upational Therapy. 2010;**4**:102-104

[26] Azma E, Safavi N. Diode laser application in soft tissue oral surgery. Journal of Lasers in Medical Science [Internet]. 2013;**4**:206-211. Available from: http://www.ncbi.nlm.nih.gov/pubmed/25606331

[27] Hend Abubaker H, Mohamad Suhaimi J, Zalila A, Zahra Al T, Farhad M, Ismail A. Influence of low power He-Ne laser irradiation on hemoglobin concentration, mean cellular volume of red blood cell, and mean cellular hemoglobin. Jurnal Sains Kesihatan Malaysia. 2011;**9**:9-13

[28] Ornitz DM, Itoh N. Fibroblast growth factors. Genome Biology [Internet]. 2001; **2**:REVIEWS3005. Available from: http://www.ncbi.nlm.nih.gov/pubmed/11276432

[29] Pang P. Lasers in cosmetic dentistry. General Dentistry. 2008;**56**:663-670

[30] Sozzi M, Fornaini C, Cucinotta A, et al. Dental ablation with 1064 nm, 500 ps, Diode pumped solid state laser: A preliminary study. Laser Therapy [Internet]. 2013;**22**(3): 195-199. Available from: http://jlc.jst.go.jp/DN/JST.JSTAGE/islsm/13-OR-16?lang=en&from=CrossRef&type=abstract

[31] Ross EV, Uebelhoer N. Laser-tissue interactions. Lasers Dermatology and Medicine. 2011:1-23

[32] Piccione PJ. Dental laser safety. Dental Clinics of North America. 2004:795-807

[33] Fornaini C, Brulat N, Milia G, et al. The use of sub-ablative Er: YAG laser irradiation in prevention of dental caries during orthodontic treatment. Laser Therapy [Internet]. 2014;**23**(3):173-181. Available from: http://www.pubmedcentral.nih.gov/articlerender.fcgi?artid=4215124&tool=pmcentrez&rendertype=abstract

[34] Staninec M, Meshkin N, Manesh SK, et al. Weakening of dentin from cracks resulting from laser irradiation. Dental Materials. 2009

[35] Miller RJ. Treatment of the contaminated implant surface using the Er,Cr:YSGG laser. Implant Dentistry. 2004

[36] Tseng W-Y, Chen M-H, Lu H-H, et al. Tensile bond strength of Er, Cr: YSGG laser-irradiated human dentin to composite inlays with two resin cements. Dental Materials Journal [Internet]. 2007;**26**:746-755. Available from: http://joi.jlc.jst.go.jp/JST.JSTAGE/dmj/26.746?from=CrossRef

Chapter 3

The Impact of Sequencing Human Genome on Drug Design to Treat Oral Cancer

Abdul Hameed Khan

Additional information is available at the end of the chapter

http://dx.doi.org/10.5772/intechopen.80231

Abstract

Of all the known cancers, oral cancer is the most preventable and it is the second most deadly cancer after the breast cancer. Out of 609,640 deaths of overall cancers, 13,500 died of oral cancer. In spite of this enormous increase in loss of life, there are no useful drugs to treat oral cancer. Sequencing human genome identifies with precision and accuracy the specific mutations responsible for causing oral cancer. In this chapter, a novel approach to design drugs to attack mutated genes in squamous cell carcinoma responsible for causing oral cancer is proposed. Alkylating aziridines attack single-stranded DNA shutting off genes. Using dinitrobenzamide dye as a carrier for aziridine, we successfully made a novel class of drugs (CB 1954) which shuts off gene of a solid tumor, Walker Carcinoma 256, in rats. We translated the animal work in humans by using quinone as a carrier for aziridines making AZQ (US Patent 4,146,622) for attacking glioblastoma for treating brain cancer in humans. We propose to search for a carrier for aziridines to attack squamous cell carcinomas to treat oral cancer. Ethical issues are discussed. Since tobacco smoking causes oral cancer, it is the most preventable disease.

Keywords: nicotine, nicotine N-oxide, aziridines, quinone, squamous cells carcinoma, glioblastoma, melphalan, pharyngeal carcinoma, nitrogen mustard, adeno-carcinoma, nitro-benzamide, nucleotide, codon, oncogene, carbamate, mitochondrial cells, AZQ

1. Historical background

Use of tobacco products will kill you. It does not matter either you smoke tobacco or you use a smokeless tobacco or nicotine patch or smoke e-cigarettes. Last year, 13,500 smokers died of oral cancer. Out of 450,000 new cancer cases diagnosed this year, 37,000 new cases will be diagnosed for 13 different types of oral cancer which include cancer of the lips, salivary glands, buccal cavity, pharynges, oropharyngeal, laryngeal, nasopharyngeal, hypopharyngeal, etc., and respiratory tract and finally lung cancers. It was Professor Ross of London University who developed oral cancer drug called melphalan (phenylalanine moiety is the carrier for the nitrogen mustard) to treat pharyngeal carcinoma [1]. Melphalan cross-links both strands of DNA shutting off genes. Statistics is worst for smokers. Over 155,700 Americans died of lung cancer last year and over 222,500 will be diagnosed this year. Compare the US mortality, the worldwide figure is ten times as high. While squamous cell carcinoma is responsible for causing oral cancer, adenocarcinoma is one of the deadliest forms of lung cancers. Most patients die within 5 years of their diagnosis. Tobacco smoking kills faster.

For years, we have been trying to answer three important questions: What is cancer? What causes cancer? And how could we diagnosed treat and prevent cancer. For this chapter, I have divided my presentation in three parts. First, I will provide some historical background; second, I will describe how efforts are being made to develop novel drugs to treat cancer; and finally, I will share some ethical problems we are facing today.

Today, we must tell all smokers in the world that tobacco smoking whether it is the regular cigarette or e-cigarette or nicotine patch or the use of smokeless tobacco, and all tobacco modifications contains nicotine, and it is the nicotine which causes oral and lung cancers. If you are diagnosed with lung cancer, you are most likely to die within 5 years. Tobacco companies have known this fact for more than half a century. In the late 1930s, German scientists discovered the fact that tobacco tar causes lung cancer [2]. When Adolf Hitler was elected as the Chancellor of Germany, he authorized 100,000 Deutsch Marks to a science research institute in Munich to isolate and identify all components of tobacco tar which causes lung cancer. He ordered all his uniform officers including pregnant women not to smoke tobacco. These facts are still available in the National archive. Tobacco companies are aware of these facts. For the past 60 years, tobacco companies have lied to us. No one was spending more money on tobacco research than tobacco companies themselves and yet when they confirmed German's finding in early 1960s that smoking causes lung cancer, they hid the fact from general public. For almost 50 years, the greedy tobacco companies exposed millions of smokers around the world with thousands of deadly chemicals with disastrous consequences. Up to this time, more than 6000 toxic chemicals have been isolated and identified from tobacco tar and 60 of those chemicals are deadly and known to cause cancer. The main constituent of tobacco tar nicotine is one of the most addictive chemicals isolated and is probably more addictive than opium. In India, the second most populous nation on Earth, last year, of the 1 million people who died of cancer, almost a quarter million died of lung cancer. Last year alone, about 3 million people died of lung cancer around the world. By the year 2020, smoking will most likely kill about 10 million people worldwide. Most smokers will prematurely die in their middle ages, cutting 20–25 years from their life expectancy. If we examine the death rate during the last 48 years, from 1950 to 1998, you will be shocked to learn that about 50 million men and 10 million women died of cancers by tobacco smoking and related illnesses.

The tobacco companies have flooded so much money in the Congressional and Senatorial election campaign, in the US alone, the US senate had voted not to ban tobacco sale to school-aged teenagers. Greedy tobacco executives won the day and needy millions around the world lost the day. Now, tobacco companies will be exporting over 150 billion cigarettes per year to the Asian continent particularly targeting India and China where almost half of the world's population live. It is a sad day for all of us. The young people, who are getting addicted to smoking today, will start dying 20 years from now. Of all cancers, tobacco smoking remains the single major preventable cause of cancer deaths in the world.

2. What is cancer?

Cancer is a very ancient disease. The early Greek coined the term cancer. They thought that this unusual disease spread like a crab so they were the first to call it a cancer or crab. The answer to the first question is that cancer is the abnormal growth of the normal cells due to accumulation of mutations over lifetime.

Our body is made of about 100 trillion cells. These cells are constantly being replaced by similar young fresh cells. For example, your white blood cells (WBCs) live for about 120 days. They are replaced by other white blood cells. Liver cells make more liver cells and replace old liver cells with new liver cells; lung cells make new lung cells. When this normal cell regulation breaks down, liver cells do not produce liver cells; they produce altered cells called mutant cells. Mutation is caused by exposure to radiations, chemical pollutions, viral infection, or genetic inheritance. The changed cells grow much faster than the normal cells and they form a lump, we call it a tumor. As tumor grows, it spreads over to the nearby blood circulating vessels. When tumor grows over these vessels, it draws more nourishment than the normal cells. Some of the tumor cells break off and split and plunge in the blood stream. These live tumor cells flow in the blood stream and travel wherever the blood goes. If the blood goes to the brain, the free floating tumor cells deposit in the brain and start growing as the brain tumors called metastasized cells. Although the cancer may have started in the lungs from smoking, it may spread to the brain or to other organs of our body. Only cancer cells spread this way; we call these migratory deposits metastasized cells, and only metastasized cells invade neighboring organs causing spread of cancer. We have no cure against metastasized cancers.

How many kinds of cancers do we have? There is a cancer for every tissue type in our body. There are 220 types of tissues in our body. Every tissue type in our body can suffer from cancer because every tissue in our body is replaced cells by cells with younger cells; they can either be replaced by normal cells in healthy people or they can also be replaced by abnormal or mutated cells when we get cancer. Would you believe that even your bones are being replaced? You could also get bone cancer.

3. What causes cancer?

Short answer is exposure to radiations, chemical pollutants like smoking, viral infection, or genetic inheritance. This is the most important question and I want to spend more time explaining the causes of cancer. This is where we spent most of the $30 billion during the lasts 30 years trying to understand how normal cells become abnormal. If we understand how they become abnormal, we should be able to treat them.

In 1971, President Richard Nixon declared war on cancer and released hundreds of millions of dollars for cancer research. He challenged Americans, the way President John Kennedy had challenged Americans a decade earlier to land men on the moon and bring them back safely. Although both presidents had great ideas, but there was a major difference.

At the time President Kennedy made that famous speech in the US congress, most of the engineering problems had already been worked out. For example, we already knew the engine thrust and its lift off power needed to leave Earth's gravity. It was calculated to be 7 miles/minute or burning fuel in the absence of air to excel the spacecraft. These engineering problems had already been solved and the knowledge was already available. Only money and trained men power were needed to build the spacecrafts. Within 10 years of that speech, President Kennedy's dream was turned to reality. On July 20, 1969, Americans landed men on the moon and brought them back safely.

But when President Nixon declared war on cancer, money was made available, but the knowledge was not there. We did not exactly know the inner working of a single living cell and how a normal cell functions, and we did not know why the normal cell becomes abnormal or cancerous. Some basic knowledge was available. In 1953, the big discovery was made in Cambridge University, England. Crick and Watson had determined the double helical structure of the genetic material DNA and postulated how the living cells divide and cells grow, and they were awarded Nobel Prize for their discovery [3]. Armed with this knowledge, we were ready to understand how a normal cell functions. Crick and Watson also opened the doors for the Nobel Prize Club. Every year, since then, a new Nobel Laureate was added to the genetic club. Soon after, Marshall Nirenberg broke the genetic code and unlocked the secret of life by showing that only three nucleotides code for an amino acid, the building block of protein. The remaining codes were deciphered by Salvador Ochoa, followed by an Indian Scientist, Govind Khorana who shared the Nobel Prize with Walter Gilbert.

After President Nixon's speech, it had taken about 20 years to understand how a normal cell functions and how it becomes abnormal by exposure to radiations, chemical pollutants, viral infection, or genetic inheritance. Let me summarize below the work of a dozen Nobel Laureates: To understand cancer, you have to understand how a normal cell functions and how it becomes abnormal. We made step by step progress over the past 30 years. First, you might ask why we study a single cell and why a single cell is so important. The fact is our life begins with a single cell. You and I are the loving union of our parents. Both parents contribute half the genetic material to each cell. Our father contributed one sperm and our mother contributed one egg. When the egg and sperm join together, we were conceived. We grow as a single cell in our mother's womb. This single cell has a set of complete instructions to construct us within in 9 months. By the time we are grown up to adulthood, that single cell makes over 100 trillion copies of itself.

During replication, if we introduce slight error in the nucleotide sequence called mutation by exposing to radiations or chemical pollutants including nicotine, viral infection, or genetic inheritance, the error is copied in every other cell. At this stage, pregnant mothers should be extremely careful what they eat and what they drink and to avoid exposing the fetus from the secondhand smokers and should stay away from smokers as far as they could. Every cell in our body has a complete library of our genome and carries complete instructions to make our brain, our nose, our ears, our arms, and our legs. Although each cell carries complete instructions to make all the organs, not all cells make all organs, but each cell begins to receive specific instructions to take a different role as it begins to make more copies. We call this process the cell differentiation.

3.1. Mutations

Damage to DNA nucleotide called mutations produces disastrous change in the information molecules. As I said above, mutations are caused by exposure to radiations, chemical pollution, viral infection, or genetic inheritance. In addition to hundreds of chemicals isolated from tobacco tar, the most potent carcinogen is nicotine N-oxide. As mutation begins in a single biological molecule, it is called a point mutation. To study changes in genetic profile of a single cell, we examine the entire genome of the same single cell. As cells grow rapidly, other mistakes in DNA replications are most likely to occur such as deletion, insertion, or inversions of nucleotide sequence. Such additional mutations are responsible for causing major diseases. Before the completion of Human Genome Project, NCI screened thousands of chemicals, plant extracts, and animal extracts for their antitumor activity. By trial and error, one in several thousand turned out to be useful. There was a need to make a rational approach to design drugs.

In 1990, United State Congress authorized 3 billion dollars to NIH to decipher the entire human genome within 15 years that is the total genetic information that makes us human called the Human Genome Project. Thousands of scientists from 6 industrialized nations and 20 biomedical centers joined our effort, and within 13 years, the entire human genome was deciphered and published in the scientific journal *Nature* [4–8] and linked to website. If you have an access to a computer keyboard, you have access to all that information.

On April 3, 2003, we read the Human Genome, the entire book of life. We found that less than 2% of the genome codes for proteins and the rest is the noncoding region which contains switches to turn the genes on or off. We can cut and paste genetic letters in the noncoding region which could serve as markers and which has no effect, but a slight change in the coding region makes a normal cell abnormal or cancerous.

A single cell is so small that we cannot even see with our naked eyes. We have to use a powerful microscope to enlarge its internal structure. Under an electron microscope, we can enlarge that one cell up to nearly a million times of its original size. Under the electron microscope, a single cell looks as big as our house. There is a good metaphor with our house. For example, our house has a kitchen, the cell has a nucleus. Imagine for a moment that our kitchen has 23 volumes of cookbooks which contain 24,000 recipes to make different dishes for our breakfast, lunch, and dinner. The nucleus has 23 pairs of chromosomes which contain 24,000 genes which carry instructions to make proteins. Proteins interact to make cells; cells interact to make tissues; and tissues interact to make an organ and several organs interact to make a man, a mouse, or a monkey. In every cell of our body, we carry 16,000 good genes, 6000 mutated genes responsible for 6000 diseases, and 2000 pseudogenes that have lost their functions, during evolutionary time.

Our entire book of life is written in four letters, and they are A (adenine), T (thymine), G (guanine), and C (cytosine). These four chemicals are called nucleotide and they are found in the nucleus of all living cells including humans, plants, and animals. Instruction in a single gene is written in thousands of AT/GC base pairs that are linked together in a straight line and we call them DNA (deoxyribonucleic acid—Nobel prize was awarded to Crick and Watson for describing the double helical nature of the DNA structure). When thousands to millions of AT/GC base pairs contain information to make a single protein, we call that portion of AT/GC base pairs a gene (Nobel Prize was awarded to Khorana and Gilbert for making a functional gene). The genes begin to function with a start codon (AUG) and stop working at the following three stop codon: UGA, UGG, and UAG. After the stop codon, no more amino acids are added and DNA synthesis stops. If we count all the AT/GC base pairs in a single cell of our body, we will find that there are 3.2 billion pairs present in every cell. The entire AT/GC sequence of 3.2 billion base pair is called the human genome or the book of our life which carries total genetic information to make us.

We deciphered all 46 chromosomes. What surprises us most is that our genome contains 6,400,000,000 nucleotide bases, half from our father and half from our mother. Less than 2% of our genome contains genes which code for proteins. The other 98% of our genome contains switches, promoters, terminators, etc. The 46 chromosomes present in each cell of our body are the greatest library of the human book of life on planet Earth. The chromosomes carry genes which are written in nucleotides. Before sequencing (determining the number and the order of the four nucleotides on a chromosome), it is essential to know how many genes are present on each chromosome in our genome. The Human Genome Project has identified the following genes on each chromosome. We found that the chromosome (1) is the largest chromosome carrying 263 million A, T, G, and C nucleotide bases and has only 2610 genes. The chromosome (2) contains 255 million nucleotide bases and has only 1748 genes. The chromosome (3) contains 214 million nucleotide bases and carries 1381 genes. The chromosome (4) contains 203 million nucleotide bases and carries 1024 genes. The chromosome (5) contains 194 million nucleotide bases and carries 1190 genes. The chromosome (6) contains 183 million nucleotide bases and carries 1394 genes. The chromosome (7) contains 171 million nucleotide bases and carries 1378 genes. The chromosome (8) contains 155 million nucleotide bases and carries 927 genes. The chromosome (9) contains 145 million nucleotide bases and carries 1076 genes. The chromosome (10) contains 144 million nucleotide bases and carries 983 genes. The chromosome (11) contains 144 million nucleotide bases and carries 1692 genes. The chromosome (12) contains 143 million nucleotide bases and carries 1268 genes. The chromosome (13) contains 114 million nucleotide bases and carries 496 genes. The chromosome (14) contains 109 million nucleotide bases and carries 1173 genes. The chromosome (15) contains 106 million nucleotide bases and carries 906 genes. The chromosome (16) contains 98 million nucleotide bases and carries 1032 genes. The chromosome (17) contains 92 million nucleotide bases and carries 1394 genes. The chromosome (18) contains 85 million nucleotide bases and carries 400 genes. The chromosome (19) contains 67 million nucleotide bases and carries 1592 genes. The chromosome (20) contains 72 million nucleotide bases and carries 710 genes. The chromosome (21) contains 50 million nucleotide bases and carries 337 genes. Finally, the sex chromosome of all female called the (X) contains 164 million nucleotide bases and carries 1141 genes. The male sperm chromosome (Y) contains 59 million nucleotide bases and carries 255 genes.

If you add up all genes in the 23 pairs of chromosomes, they come up to 26,808 genes and yet we keep on mentioning 24,000 genes. The remaining genes are called the pseudogenes. For example, millions of years ago, humans and dog shared some of the same ancestral genes; we both carry the same olfactory genes. Since humans do not use these genes to smell for searching food, these genes are broken and they lose their functions in humans, but we still carry them. We call them pseudogenes. Recently, some Japanese scientists have activated the pseudogenes; this work may create ethical problem in future as more and more pseudogenes are activated.

The above DNA nucleotide bases constitute the genetic map of the normal human being; what makes them abnormal and makes us sick is the mutation in the coding regions of the genome. Now, we can examine the tumor genome of the oral cancer patients to identify specific mutations responsible for causing the disease. As I said above, less than 2% of the genome codes for amino acids. Slightest damage to the coding regions of the four nucleotides A, T, G, and C either by radiations, chemical pollution (from tobacco tar), genetic inheritance, or viral infection or by insertion, deletion, or inversion of the nucleotide bases code for wrong or abnormal amino acids resulting in diseases.

Although you and I are both human and yet no two individuals look the same because the AT/GC base pairs in each of us are arranged slightly differently, a difference of one nucleotide in a thousand base pair. The amazing fact is that out of 3,000,000,000 AT/GC base pairs, only 3 pairs of AT/GC code for a single amino acid, the building blocks of protein, called a codon (Nobel Prize was awarded to Nierenberg and Ochoa). Codons are the most important collections of AT/GC base pairs because they have correct instructions to make the right amino acids (there are only 20 amino acids; they randomly combine to make a protein). Thousands of amino acids make a protein and thousands of proteins make a cell; billions of cells make a tissue and hundreds of tissues make an organ and several organs make an individual such as you and me. This is how normal cell functions and we begin to grow.

As I said above, the old cells begin to die and they are constantly being replaced by healthy cells. Why do the normal cells become abnormal or become cancerous? Any factor that disrupts the 2% of the coding region of our genome will alter its function by slightly altering its code; an altered codon will code for a wrong amino acid and a wrong amino acid will give a wrong protein and it will make normal cell abnormal. When the functions of codons are disrupted intentionally or unintentionally, we alter the codon's function. For example, intentionally we alter a codon by smoking and unintentionally by exposure to environmental pollution such as chemicals or radiations. Altered codons have wrong information to make wrong amino acids. Wrong amino acids make wrong proteins and wrong proteins make wrong cells and wrong cells grow much faster than the normal cells and become abnormal or cancerous and they form a lump, we call these lumps tumors.

Four factors will disrupt a codon's function. Two are minor such as viruses and inherited oncogenes, and two are major such as radiations and chemical pollutants in our environment. Let me explain how a codon is altered:

3.1.1. Virus

HPV causes more than 32,000 cases of cancer including oral cancer every year in the US. It is also very preventable by giving HPV vaccine for children at ages 11–12 which can protect them.

Viruses are not considered germ in the classical sense because they lack the ability to reproduce its progeny independently. To reproduce their own kind, viruses attack DNA of living cells, whether they are humans, animals, or plant cells. Viruses are also fragments of DNA that have the ability to merge in the host cell DNA and become integrated and invisible. They infect (merge) host's DNA and alter its functional machinery in such a way as to make protein and progeny for themselves. Not all viruses are bad. If all viruses kill their host cells, they will die too. Only a handful of virulent viruses destroy host cells. For example, AIDS viruses in human disrupt the codons and cause a unique cancer in AIDS patients called Kaposi carcinoma. Hardly anyone survives that cancer.

3.1.2. Oncogene

Oncogenes are also fragments of mutated DNA, but they are always bad. They are complete genes that have the instructions to make a specific bad protein. Such genes are called oncogenes (cancer-causing genes). Our institute's, NIH's, past Director, Dr. Harold Varmus, was the first man to identify an oncogene in humans. For his work, Dr. Varmus shared a Nobel Prize with Dr. Michael Bishop.

From here begins one of the most exciting stories that explain the causes of cancer. In the early 1990s, some scientists in England were studying cancer-causing viruses. When scientists injected cancer-causing viruses to animals, they found that sometimes viruses grow and other times they do not. On close examination, they detected a background protein in all cells. Whenever the background protein is absent, cancer-causing viruses grow and the animal develops cancer. Whenever the background protein is present, cancer-causing viruses will not grow. They called it the background Protein 53 or (P53). They identify the gene that makes P53 protein and they named P53 gene. Since cancer is suppressed in the presence of P53, scientists named P53 as cancer suppressor proteins. When a normal cell is damaged, the surrounding cells grow to make P53 protein to repair the damage. When healing is complete, the P53 protein stops the cells from further growth. If there is a mutation in the P53 gene, P53 loses its function and the cell growth will not stop and grow continuously and become cancerous.

As I said above, that gene is a collection of codons and each codon is made of three pairs of AT/GC. Hundreds of thousands to millions of AT/GC base pairs combine to form gene-53. Now, we know that the codon in P53 is sensitive to mutation by chemicals, radiations, viruses, and oncogenes. If you cause a slight defect in the codon by altering one letter of AT/GC base pair, the entire P53 gene becomes defected. Defected P53 cannot produce background protein that suppresses cancer. In the absence of P53 protein, patients develop cancer. The lesson we learn is that if a single letter of this four-letter AT/GC base pairs is altered by virus or by chemicals or by gene or by radiation, first a single normal cell becomes abnormal or cancerous. Over many replications, the mutated cell becomes cancerous. Repeated exposure to chemicals such as smoking tobacco several times a day, you could alter a single letter of AT/GC base pairs. If a single cell becomes defected, it will multiply and accumulate and an entire organ becomes cancerous. When the defected organ cannot function, we become ill.

Unfortunately, cancer is not localized at one place for long (we could have cut out the defected organ and throw it away); it spreads or metastasizes as I described above. Once it is metastasized, the other organs lose their function; with too many defected organs, a patient cannot survive for long. When we examine the internal structure of tumors of a dead patient, we find it mostly consists of abnormal cells that have been altered.

Let me tell you what you can do to protect yourselves and what we can do to help you? If you want to protect yourselves from oral or lung cancers, stop taking tobacco in any form and in any kind. The best way we can help you is to pursue as vigorously as we could do to find other sensitive genes and try to replace them with healthy genes by a method called gene therapy. Gene therapy could work if a single gene is mutated. Unfortunately, several genes are mutated in oral lung cancers. Gene therapy fails, but drug therapy works. From here my work begins. Professor Ross and I design drugs to shut off multiple defected genes.

As I said above, although the book of life is written in 3.2 billion AT/GC base pairs, about 2% of the AT/GC base pairs contain 24,000 genes (specific instructions to make proteins), the rest of DNA is called the junk DNA. As I said above, it is not garbage that we throw away; it contains important gene switches, promoters, enhancers, etc. We keep it because someday we might be able to find out what additional information it may provide about us. We carry all 24,000 genes in every cell of our body, but less than 6000 genes are probably bad genes (mutated) that are linked to a variety of genetic defects leading to 6000 different diseases. Each of us does not carry all 6000 bad genes, but we do carry a single copy of at least 4–5 bad genes in our genome. They remain dormant because only one parent carries a single copy of a mutated gene. We need both bad copies of bad genes, one from each parent to get sick. We have inherited these bad genes from our parents. Our parents inherited these genes from their parents. One ancestor can pass on the same bad genes to her children and children's children. Therefore, it is a wise idea not to marry within the same family tree. The more intermarriages among the same family members, the more bad genes tend to concentrate among fewer and fewer children of that family.

3.1.3. Nicotine N-oxide is a carcinogen

I could take tobacco extract samples to the lab and analyze its ingredients. First, I soak the tobacco in ammonia and extract with chloroform. All nitrogen bases are extracted in chloroform. I could wash the extract with water to remove all water-soluble impurities and dry the extract and distill off the chloroform. I place the residue in long glass column filled with silica gel. I pour a solvent mixture which carries the residue down the column. It is called the separation of different components by chromatography. I shine the UV light on the glass column as the solvent flows down. Hundreds of different bands appear in different colors, corresponding to hundreds of components present in the tobacco tar. The largest band is nicotine. To confirm, I take a little sample from the band and inject in the MS (mass spectrometer: the largest peak corresponds to the molecular weight of the nicotine). I could make the radiolabeled nicotine by adding C-14 diazomethane in sodium hydroxide. The reaction adds a radiolabeled methyl group to nicotine molecule. I inject the radiolabeled methyl nicotine to half a dozen mice. I collect their urine samples separately. Analysis of the urine sample shows that some mice produce no change and others produce a new chemical called nicotine N-oxide. All those mice in which the gene that produces monoamine oxidase was activated developed cancer. If you inject nicotine N-oxide to another set of a dozen mice, they all come down with various cancers. All aromatic N-oxides are carcinogens.

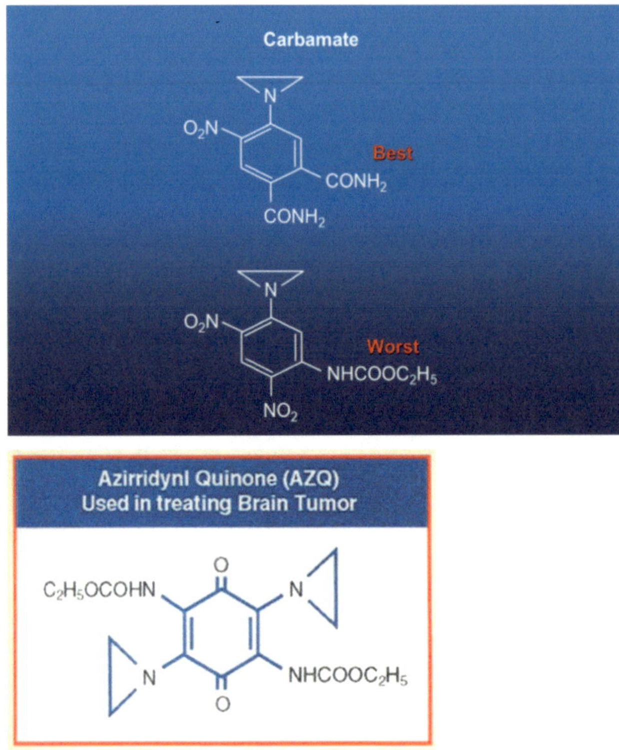

Figure 1. NIH Scientific Achievement Award. Aziridines as single strand DNA binding agent.

Now, you know why Sir Winston Churchill, who smoked cigar all his life, never developed cancer, but film actor Yul Brenner smoked cigarettes and died of lung cancer. If you were to analyze their urine samples, you will find that Mr. Brenner urine contains nicotine N-oxide. The gene monoamine oxidase is activated in Brenner to make nicotine N-oxide not in Sir Winston. While Sir Winston lived, Brenner died.

While I was busy designing drugs, such as AZQ, to shut off genes which cause brain cancers, my colleagues in the other labs at NCI (National Cancer Institute) have isolated hundreds of chemicals from the tobacco tar which contains dozens of carcinogenic chemicals. If you would apply the tobacco tar on the skin of mice, within a few weeks, tumor develops on the skin surface. The major culprit is nicotine which is considered as one of the most addictive chemicals. Some studies showed that it is even more addictive than many known narcotics such as marijuana, opiates, and heroin. Oral cancer (OC) is caused by chemicals released by chewing tobacco. Most football players chew tobacco; they call it smokeless tobacco. Smoking burns tobacco generating even more aromatic amines which are known carcinogens. Nitrosoamines bind to DNA producing mutations.

After the completion of the Human Genome Project, we have identified specific mutations responsible for a specific disease. Now, we design drugs to attack that specific mutation to shut off that gene. The completion of the Human Genome Project has the greatest impact on developing drugs on a rational basis and for treating various cancers including the oral cancer. The technologies developed during the completion of the Human Genome Project (the tool kits which contain hundreds of restrictions enzymes to cut DNA ligase to join DNA pieces; using these tool kits, we can cut, paste, and copy genes) could be used to treat and prevent oral cancer. The recently completed Thousand Genome Project will pinpoint with precision and accuracy the specific damage to DNA nucleotides responsible for causing various oral cancers. Once the mutated genes on a specific chromosome are identified, we can design drugs to shut off those genes like we designed AZQ (US Patent 4,146,622) to attack brain tumor (for structure, see **Figure 1**).

Once the mutation sites and chromosome numbers are identified, we can diagnose, prevent, and treat the oral cancer either by gene therapy if a single gene mutation is responsible for causing any of the above cancers or by drug therapy if multiple mutations are involved. As I stated above, French Anderson and his colleagues have successfully developed gene therapy for treating SCID (severe combined immunodeficiency) syndrome; we could use the same method to cut and paste and replace the bad gene with the good gene in a virus which is used to infect the WBC obtained from the same patient. After harvesting the infected WBC, the transgenic WBC was injected back in the same patient to treat SCID. It worked and patients fully recovered. Several thousand SCID children are living a normal life. Gene therapy works with a single gene mutation, but not if the multiple mutations are responsible for causing diseases.

4. Historical background for drug design

On the other hand, if cancer is caused by multiple mutations, we could use drug therapy by preventing malignant cell replication developed by Ross by cross-linking both strands of DNA. Using dyes specific to OC cells as carriers for nitrogen mustard, as done by Ross in making Melphalan, we could also develop new class of drugs to attack cancer cells in the other parts of the oral cavity. The bad news is that there have been 13 different forms of oral cancer identified. The good news is that for designing a drug, we have to find a dye which colors one of these tumors. There are hundreds of dyes available for testing. Once we succeed in finding a dye, we could design drugs by using our method by attaching aziridines to attack that specific oral cancer by shutting off mutated genes by binding to a single strand of DNA. What would happen if we succeed and when next-generation sequencers produce inexpensive and fast sequencing genomes is that we could identify all mutated genes on all 13 oral cancers with precision and accuracy and design drugs to shut off those genes.

In the laboratory of the Sir Walter Ross at the Royal Cancer Hospital of London University, England, I was trained to design drugs to attack mutated DNA shutting off mutated genes. Professor Ross had spent all his life working on "Biological Alkylating Agents" and published a series of paper including a book [9–13]. Using the same rationale, I worked with Professor Ross for almost 10 years at London University developing anticancer drugs. Instead of cross-linking DNA with nitrogen mustards, I used aziridines to bind to a single strand of DNA shutting off the genes.

During 10-year period in the Professor Ross' Lab, I made over 120 such drugs to attack a solid tumor called the Walker carcinoma 256 in rats. The most effective drug was called CB 1954 (2-4, dinitrophenyl aziridinyl benzamide) (see structure in **Figure 1**). It was 70 times more toxic to the tumor cell [14]. It is the most effective drug ever made against the solid experimental tumor for which I was honored with the Royal Cancer Hospital's Institute Cancer Research postdoctoral award. Why mutated DNA must be attacked is because mutated DNAs code for wrong amino acids which produce wrong protein and cause abnormal growth leading to cancers. The reason why we work on mouse model is that if you would compare the genome of man, mouse, and monkey, they are all mammalians and their genomes are very similar. Once you succeed in attacking mouse tumor, it opens gate to attack human tumors. Now, you know how challenging it is to shutting off a mutated gene and how easy it is to introduce mutations in the same gene by smoking.

The good news about smokers is that they could see their own genome on their computers and could also see the progress of mutations of their own genomes before and after smoking. Now, I do not have to tell my best friends not to smoke. All I have to do is to give the two CDs of their genomes and let them see for themselves. Let them see on their own computers and compare the two genomes. First, CD taken soon after their birth and second taken after they become smokers. Before I talk about the sequence-specific tumors of oral and lung cancers, let me share with you how our genome, the book of our life, looks like before you smoke.

The basis of OC is that people who are chewing tobacco or inhaling burning tobacco by smoking (as in India) or chewing betel quid, betel nut, etc. (as in Taiwan) causing major mutations in their genomes producing a host of chemicals which damage the normal function of the cell causing them to become abnormal or cancerous. To understand the molecular basis of cancers, we have to sequence the normal as well as cancer cell genomes for comparison.

To refresh your memory, I repeat. Carcinoma is the most common type of cancer. It begins in the epithelial tissue of the skin, or in the tissue that lines the internal organs, such as mouth, oral cavity, reparatory tract, and lungs. There are 220 different types of tissues in the normal human being. We have sequenced (read letter by letter the entire script of nucleotides, their numbers, and their orders in which they are arranged). After genome sequencing, we can compare with the sequence of oropharynx carcinoma with normal cell from nonsmokers. I am happy to inform you that we just completed the Thousand Genome Project. Now, we can compare thousands of the same mutated sequence a time. We can locate the specific mutations with precision and accuracy. To locate specific mutations, in all oral cavity cancers, similar comparison can be studied in several types of salivary gland cancers including adenoid cystic carcinoma, mucoepidermoid carcinoma, and polymorphous low-grade adenocarcinoma. Tonsils and base of the tongue tissues also develop lymphomas.

Once a mutation is identified in a specific oral cancer, my job begins trying to find a dye which colors these tumors. Once a dye is found, I could attach the toxic groups to shut off their genes. There are hundreds of dyes and there are hundreds of their combinations. With AT and GC, four nucleotides of DNA, I get 64 combinations; imagine how many combinations I get from hundreds of dyes. Fortunately, there are finite combinations. I could find it. Suppose I want to design drugs to treat cancers of the oral cavity. The cancer begins in the epithelial tissue of the skin, or in the tissue that lines the internal organs, such as mouth, oral cavity, reparatory tract, and finally reaching lungs. We have been designing drugs to attack toughest solid tumor like

http://dx.doi.org/10.5772/intechopen.80231

Walker carcinoma 256 in rats or glioblastoma in humans. It would be much easier to attack carcinoma. And also suppose that I find a single dye which specifically colors a specific carcinoma cell. Now, my work begins to attach aziridines or carbamate or both as we succeeded in making AZQ for attacking brain tumor. Nowadays, I have to submit the research proposal to the Safety Committee (IRB: Institutional Review Board) for their approval. Since I will be using highly toxic nerve gases and nitrogen mustard, the proposal will be rejected.

5. Drug design for treating cancer

Firtz Heber, a German Army officer, worked on the development of chemicals as a weapon of war. He was responsible for making deadly nerve gases and nitrogen mustards. Before the WWI, he was honored with a Nobel Prize for capturing nitrogen directly from the atmosphere by burning the element magnesium in the air forming its nitride. Upon hydrolysis, nitride is converted to its nitrate which is used as a fertilizer. Using this method, we could make unlimited amount fertilizer. Nitrate is also used for making explosive. Soon after the WWI, Heber was charged with a crime against humanity for releasing hundreds of cylinders of chlorine gas on the Western front killing thousands of soldiers in the trenches. When allied forces reached his residence, his son shot himself and his wife committed suicide. Heber went in hiding in Switzerland. After the war, German government got his release as a part of the peace negotiations. Heber returned home to hero's welcome. Although he promised never to work on the nerve gases again, secretly he continued to develop more lethal analogs of highly toxic nitrogen mustards. It was Heber who first made the notorious bis-dichloroethyl methyl amine. Because it smells like mustard seeds, it is called as nitrogen mustard. During the next 20 years, before the beginning of the WWII, hundreds of more toxic analogs of nitrogen mustard were developed. The bad news is that they are highly toxic and the good news is that they shut off genes.

6. Rationale for developing anticancer drugs

Nitrogen mustard was mercilessly used during the WWII by both German and Italian armies against allied forces. Most soldiers exposed to nitrogen mustard were frozen to death. Their blood analysis showed a sharp decline in white blood cell (WBC). Since patients with the cancer of the blood called leukemia showed a sharp increase of WBC, Professor Ross and his group wondered if minimum amount of nitrogen mustard could be used to control leukemia in cancer patients. It was a success. For the following 30 years, Ross developed hundreds of derivatives of nitrogen mustard to treat a variety of cancers. His most successful drugs are chlorambucil, melphalan, and merophan [2–6, 14].

Radiolabeled study showed that nitrogen mustard shut off genes by binding to DNA by cross-linking. At London University, I work for Professor Ross for almost 10 years first as his graduate student, then his post-doctoral fellow, and then as his special assistant. I worked with the deadliest nerve agents such as nitrogen mustards, carbamates, and aziridines developed during Hitler's time for evil purposes. We are converting evil into good. These agents easily pass through various layers of our skin from ectoderm to mesoderm to endoderm. They easily enter the cell nucleus destroying the beta and gamma cell which develop immunity. Then they enter the nuclear membrane where they find the stem cells. Stem cells differ from say skin cells. In stem cells, all 24,000 genes are functioning and they have not yet differentiated, but skin cells are differentiated and they have shut off all other genes except the skin cell genes.

To the above toxic agents, I attach dyes to attack one of the carcinoma cells. The toxic group is activated by cell's enzyme to produce a positive carbon ion called carbonium ion. It is extremely reactive; it binds to all four nucleotides (AT and GC) which form the DNA. But it preferentially binds to N-7 of guanine killing the stem cells. Professor Ross and I have demonstrated the attack on N-7 of guanine using the radiolabeled study.

If I am accidentally exposed to any of the above toxic agents, I do not die of mustard poisoning; I would be frozen to death. What happens is the following: each cell carries hundreds of mitochondrial cells (mitochondria are foreign cells called prokaryotes without nuclear membrane captured by human cells during the evolutionary period, millions of years ago; they live in symbiotic relationship; to perform daily function, mitochondria provide energy to human cells and human cells provide free food and free housing to the mitochondria) which carry energy-rich phosphate bonds. They produce energy by breaking phosphate bonds in which a chemical called ATP (adenosine triphosphate) is broken down to ADP (adenosine diphosphate) which is further broken down to AMP (adenosine monophosphate). As normal cell grows, an enzyme attaches inorganic phosphate to the AMP regenerating ATP. If mitochondrial cells die, there is no energy available.

As I said above, NIH is the largest biomedical center in the world. It has unlimited facilities (chemicals, equipment, and personnel). Twenty-one thousand best and brightest scientists selected from Ivy League schools work in 26 institutes in more than 3000 labs. I had sent NIH over 120 drugs for NCI screening program [14–16]. During the 3-year period at NIH labs, I

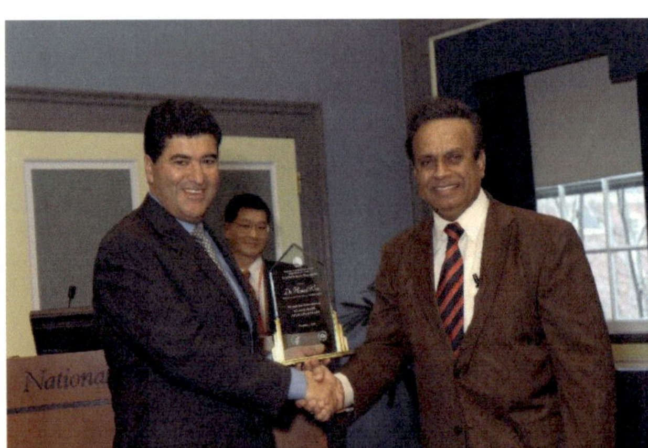

Figure 2. 2004 NIH Scientific Achievement Award presented to Dr. Hameed Khan by Dr. Elias Zerhouni, the Director of NIH during the NIH/APAO award ceremony held on December 3, 2004. Dr. Khan is the discoverer of AZQ (US Patent 4,146,622), a novel experimental drug specifically designed to shut off a gene that causes brain cancer for which he receives a 17-year royalty for his invention (License Number L-0I9-0I/0). To this date, more than 300 research papers have been published on AZQ. The award ceremony was broadcast live worldwide by the Voice of America (VOA). Dr. Khan is the first Indian to receive one of the America's highest awards in Medicine.

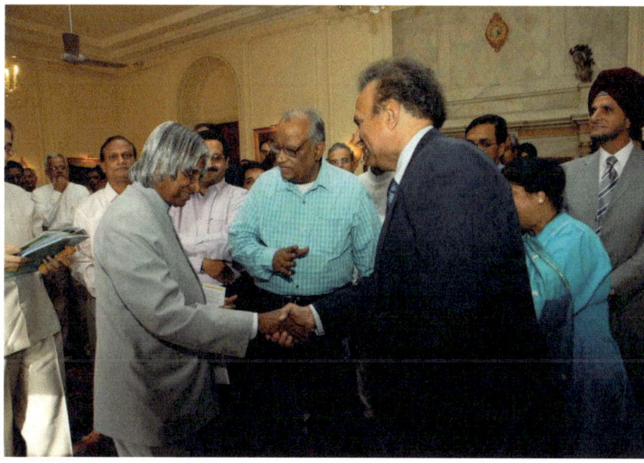

Figure 3. His excellency, Dr. A.P.J. Abdul Kalam, the President of India greeting Dr. A. Hameed Khan, discoverer of anticancer AZQ, after receiving 2004, Vaidya Ratna, the Gold Medal, one of the India's highest awards in medicine at the Rashtrapathi Bhavan (Presidential Palace), in Delhi, India, during a reception held on April 2, 2004.

made AZQ (US Patent 4,146,622) and 45 patentable analogs [17–19]. Years later, I was honored for my work on developing AZQ. Almost 20 years later, for translating my work from mouse to man and making AZQ (US Patent 4,146,622) for treating brain cancer, I was honored with the "2004 NIH Scientific Achievement Award," one of the America's highest awards in medicine (**Figure 2**). I was also honored by the Government of India with Vaidya Ratna (Gold Medal) (**Figure 3**).

In spite of all the risks, fear, and challenges, the zeal and the enthusiasm that I had to design drugs to attack brain cancer like AZQ is not there to treat oral or lung cancers. Do you know why because I know in my heart, the patient once cured will go back to smoking again. He cannot help it; it is an addiction (**Figure 4**) [20, 21].

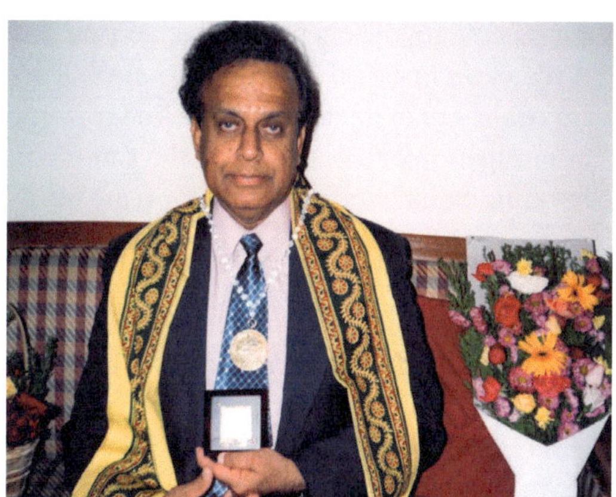

Figure 4. Gold Medal for Dr. Khan. Dr. A. Hameed Khan, a scientist at the National Institutes of Health (NIH), USA, and an American Scientist of Indian origin, was awarded on April 2, 2004. Vaidya Ratna, the Gold Medal, one of the India's highest awards in medicine for his discovery of AZQ (US Patent 4,146,622) which is now undergoing clinical trials for treating brain cancer.

7. Forbidden area

Firtz Haber was a hero to some for getting a Nobel Prize for capturing nitrogen directly from atmosphere by burning magnesium metal in the air and hydrolyzing magnesium nitride to produce nitrate the fertilizer. To others, he was the greatest criminal because he released hundreds of cylinders of chlorine gas at the Western front killing thousands of soldiers in the trenches. It was Haber who made the nitrogen mustard and its deadly analogs which were used during WWII. Soldiers exposed to nitrogen mustard burns died of a sharp drop in the white blood cell (WBC) count. Since all cancers showed a sharp increase in WBC count, Ross decided to use modified derivatives of nitrogen mustard to control the cancer growth. Ross was successful. He attached amino acid phenylalanine as a carrier for the nitrogen mustard moiety to make melphalan for treating pharyngeal carcinoma. Over a 10-year period, I made dozens of analogs of nitrogen mustards for Ross. The deadliest among them was the phenylenediamine mustard. We use these compounds to check the sensitivity of the tumors in the tumor bank. If tumors in the tumor bank become resistant, we have to replace them with fresh more sensitive tumors for testing other compounds.

Proteins in our body are made of 20 amino acids. When Ross made melphalan by using 1 amino acid out of 20, most of my colleagues thought that they could use the following 19 amino acid to treat all 13 forms of oral cancers including lung cancer: alanine, arginine, aspartic acid, asparagine, cysteine, glycine, glutamic acid, glutamine, histidine, isoleucine, leucine, lysine, methionine, phenylalanine (Ross used this amino acid to make melphalan for treating pharyngeal carcinoma), proline, serine, threonine, tryptophan, tyrosine, and valine.

Aliphatic nitrogen mustards are deadlier than aromatic nitrogen mustards. They decided not to proceed because they do not want to risk their life to save the life of nicotine addicts. If you want to save smokes' life by risking your own, you are welcome to it. I will show you how to make the nitrogen mustard by describing Haber's crudest method. Haber reacted methylamine with ethylene oxide to make 2-bis dihydroxy ethylene methyl amine. It was chlorinated by heating with phosphorus pentachloride in the phosphoric acid. If you noticed a faint smell of mustard seed, Congratulations, you got nitrogen mustard; you are dead. No matter how much precaution you take, after the experiment, if you take an alcohol swab of walls, doors, and knobs and run mass spectra of alcohol extract, you find a line corresponding to nitrogen mustard. If you are exposed to nitrogen mustard and cross the threshold level, your WBC drops sharply and the energy-providing mitochondria die and you are most likely to freeze to death.

Will anyone approve this study, probably no one. Your IRB will reject your proposal; your safety committee will reject it and who will provide the funds for such study. No one.

Tobacco companies are rich and can afford to invest money in curing cancers. Since most of their work is conducted behind closed doors, why not make nitrogen mustard analogs of all other 19 amino acids. Like melphalan, they might find some of these analogs of amino acids of nitrogen mustard to cure oral to lung cancers. They could make money not only by giving cancers by selling tobacco products but also by treating some cancers.

8. Ethical issues

Some of my best friends smoke and most of them are not scientists. Do I tell them not to smoke and keep their friendship? Not a chance. So I tell them experimental facts as gently as possible. My readers are my best friends. All I want is to make them think. If they think, my job as a friend is done.

Scientists in our group are working on different kinds of cancers. As I stated above, there are more than 220 different types of tissues and they could all become cancerous if they are exposed to radiations or chemical environmental pollution. We are all working to cure those cancers. Unfortunately, there is no great enthusiasm for working on either oral cancer or lung cancer. Such diseases are considered self-inflicting wounds. The users of tobacco products are addicted and frequently developed these types of cancers. Many scientists believe that all of us have a free will. We have a right to live and we have a right to die. If you do not smoke or chew tobacco, you will not expose yourself to a host of carcinogens. Some of us believe that you are addicted to nicotine if we cure your oral cancer, you will go back and chew tobacco again. How can we protect you from yourself? If we protect you from yourself, we create a monster. On the other hand, if you are one of those unfortunate persons who inherit a mutated gene, or exposed to secondhand smoking or exposed to radiations or heavy metal particles, you deserve all our help and many of us have been designing drugs for treating oral and lung cancers for these innocent victims.

Author details

Abdul Hameed Khan

Address all correspondence to: hameedkhan111@comcast.net

National Center for Medical Rehabilitation Research (NCMRR), National Institutes of Health (NIH) Bethesda, MD, USA

References

[1] Ross WCJ, Mitchell M. Melphalan. Lancet. **370**(9594):1209-1218

[2] The anti-tobacco campaign of the Nazis: A little known aspect of public health in Germany, 1933-45. British Medical Journal. **313**(7070):1450-1453, 1933-1945

[3] Watson JD, Crick FHC. A structure for deoxyribose nucleic acid. Nature. 1953;**171**:737-738

[4] Nature. 2001;**409**:934-941

[5] Nature. 2001;**409**:660-921

[6] Nature. 2004;**431**:931-945

[7] Nature. 2005;**438**:803-810

[8] Nature. 2017;**550**:345-353

[9] Ross WCJ. The chemistry of cytotoxic alkylating agents. In: Greenstein JP, Haddow A, editors. Advances in Cancer Research. New York: Academic Press, Inc.; 1953. pp. 397-449

[10] Ross WCJ. Biological Alkylating Agents. London: Butterworth; 1962

[11] Ross WCJ. Journal of Chemical Society. 1949;183

[12] Ross WCJ. Journal of the Chemical Society. 1950;2257

[13] Ross WCJ, Mitchley BCV. Annual Report of the British Empire Cancer Campaign. 1964;**42**:70

[14] Cobb LM, Connors TA, Elson LA, Khan AH, Mitchley BCV, Ross WCJ, et al. 2,4-Dinitro-5-ethyleneiminobenzamide (CB 1954): A potent and selective inhibitor of the growth of the Walker Carcinoma 256. Biochemical Pharmacology. 1969;**18**:1519-1527

[15] Chlorambucil - CancerConnect News. CancerConnect News. Retrieved: 2015-12-21

[16] Hameed Khan A, Ross WCJ. Tumour-growth inhibitory nitrophenylaziridines and related compounds: Structure-activity relationships. Part I. Chemico-Biological Interactions. 1969/1970;**1**:27-47

[17] Hameed Khan A, Ross WCJ. Tumour-growth inhibitory nitrophenylaziridines and related compounds: Structure-activity relationships. PART II. Chemico-Biological Interactions. 1971/1972;**4**:11-22

[18] Hameed Khan A, Driscoll JS. Active antitumor components in a decomposed amino sugar. Part 1. Effect of sugar structure on activity. Journal of Pharmaceutical Sciences. 1975; **64**(2):295-299

[19] Hameed Khan A, Driscoll J. Potential central nervous system antitumor agents: Aziridinylbenzoquinones. Part I. Journal of Medicinal Chemistry. 1976;**19**(2):313-317

[20] Chou FT, Hameed Khan A, Driscoll J. Potential central nervous system antitumor agents: Aziridinylbenzoquinones. Part II. Journal of Medicinal Chemistry. 1976;**19**:1302

[21] Driscoll JS, Hameed Khan A, Chou F-T. Aziridinyl quinone: Anti-transplanted tumor agents. Unites States Patent # 4,146,622; March 27, 1979

Chapter 4

Early Detection and Multidisciplinary Approach to Oral Cancer Patients

Nihat Akbulut and Ahmet Altan

Additional information is available at the end of the chapter

http://dx.doi.org/10.5772/intechopen.81126

Abstract

"Oral cancer" is a term usually describing oral cavity and oropharyngeal malign tumors. The most histologic type of carcinoma is squamous cell carcinoma, seen in oral and oropharyngeal region with the incidence of 90%. Prevention or early diagnosis of premalignant and oral cancer requires increased public awareness and educating practitioners to be skillful in identifying oropharyngeal region pathology. To prevent oral cancers, the etiological factors should be known, and measures must be taken according to those factors. Premalignant lesions are leukoplakia, lichen planus in oral and cutaneous form, erythroplakia, stomatitis nicotina, and submucous fibrosis. Premalignant lesions should be treated, if possible, or followed up on carefully. To date, there are many clinical, histopathological, radiological, and optical techniques to diagnose or capture precancerous and oral cancer lesions early. The routine management of oral cancers is firstly surgical resection with or without postoperative adjuncts and other therapies such as the use of postoperative chemoradiation and radiation. Successful treatment of oral cancer patients is a complex issue that requires a multidisciplinary approach, including oral and maxillofacial surgeons, oral and maxillofacial radiologists, ENT specialists, medical and radiological oncologists, prosthodontists, dentists, speech therapists, supportive care experts, and also pathologists or, if possible, oral and maxillofacial pathologists.

Keywords: oral squamous cell carcinoma, preventive actions, early diagnosis, management of oral cancer, multidisciplinary approach, improving quality of life

1. Introduction

"Oral cancer" is a term usually used to describe oral cavity and oropharyngeal malign tumors. Oropharyngeal cancers include the regions known as buccal mucosa, hard-soft palate, and floor of mouth—gums, tonsils, and base and oral tongue remain oropharynx regions [1]. Despite this, the typical use of the term "oropharyngeal cancer" is unsuitable for this current topic due to earlier determination of "oral cancer." Although some reverse knowledge is in the literature, incidence of pharyngeal cancers is increasing, while oral cancer is declining in the USA according to the recent LeHew et al. report [1]. In addition, they connected this issue to human papillomavirus (HPV) and how it may cause many more pharyngeal cancers than oral cancers, while heavy alcohol consumption and tobacco use also cause more oral cancer. The same author emphasized ethnicity, gender, age, and other demographic factors that influence the occurrence of pharyngeal or oral cancers [1–4]. The other paper published by Yadav [2] mentioned the increase of oral or mouth cancer in young individuals, especially female individuals, and that lifestyles affect the likelihood it occurs (such as smoking or chewing tobacco, chewing betel nuts). On the other hand, lip cancer occurrence is increasing because of ozone layer loss [2].

The International Agency for Research on Cancer determined 25 years ago that types HPV 16–18 had a carcinogenic effect in humans which were responsible for the huge proportion (90%) of carcinoma of the cervix. HPV 16–18 had also been an etiologic factor related to various head, neck, and also oral carcinomas [5]. Fortunately, as relatively consolatory features of HPV-related cancers, Ang et al. [6] and Yadav [2] reported that these cancers are more sensitive to the current treatment options and have higher survival rates than other different etiologic factors, such as tobacco, causing carcinomas. Some of the other etiologic factors have mostly been seen in Southern Chinese ancestry: nasopharyngeal cancer, Epstein-Barr virus (EBV) exposure, and also consumption of salted fish [7].

Worldwide, oral cancer cases are meanly estimated at 500,000, with nearly 389,000 new cases per year and nearly 130,000 deaths [3, 4, 8]; 45,000 oral cancer cases in the USA face nearly 8500 deaths, and in the European Union, there are nearly 66,650 new cases faced each year [1, 3]. In further information found in the literature, Sri Lanka, India, Pakistan, Bangladesh, Hungary, and France show higher rates of new cases [3]. In addition to this information, South and Southeast Asian countries such as Pakistan, India, the Philippines, and Bangladesh are 80% of the newest cases due to increasing tobacco use and alcohol consumption and especially in Malaysian betel quid chewing [7–9].

The most histological type of carcinoma is squamous cell carcinoma, seen in the oral and oropharyngeal region with 90% [3, 7, 10–18]. The histological variants of squamous cell carcinomas are revealed in the literature to be adenosquamous, verrucous squamous, basaloid squamous, and papillary squamous cell carcinomas. In addition, carcinoma in situ is the previous form of the invasive squamous cell carcinomas. The other type of carcinoma of oropharyngeal mucosa in basal cells is seen rarely, in the oral cavity under 5%. On the other hand, there are many types of epithelial malignancies, such as mucoepidermoid carcinoma with 54%, low-grade adenocarcinoma with 17%, and adenoid cystic carcinoma with 15% mostly in hard palate minor salivary glands (60%), lips (25%), and vestibular mucosa (15%). Moreover, tumors being aggressive in any part of the body, mucosal melanomas are rarely seen in the hard palate and gingiva. Bony tumors, such as very rare cases of ameloblastic carcinoma, can be seen in the oral region [3]. Lymphomas and all aspects of sarcomas and odontogenic tumors, as those have a different etiology, are managed with different methods [17].

In this chapter, detection, diagnosis, multidisciplinary management, and post-management of patients with oral cancer and improvement of their quality of life will be used, instead of oral squamous cell cancer terms.

Prevention of oral cancer is an essential goal worldwide; if it is not possible to achieve this, then we should detect or diagnose oral cancer in early stages to completely manage it [1]. Prevention or early diagnosis of this entity requires public awareness action and practitioner education to be skillful in identification of oropharyngeal region pathology [4, 8].

Severity or aggression of a disease, usually termed in the literature as "stage," is essential to treating it in secure conditions without any recurrence. In addition, if it features severe aspects, it needs aggressive treatment modality such as surgical eradication and a reconstruction process. In body regions wherein cancer occurs, the classifications, severity, and level determination systems differ. The most popular system evaluating cancer type and severity is the TNM system according to two recent American Joint Committee on Cancer (AJCC) editions, the seventh and eighth [13, 19], used the world over due to its simplicity and friendly aspect [3]. The eighth edition has been in use since January, 2018. Additionally, the eighth edition differs from previous editions because it has taken HPV into account as an etiological factor [19].

In the head and neck region, the classification of cancer has been standardized with TNM levels or a stage grouping system and a histological aspect, meaning the histological grading of a disease [5, 20]. Oral cancers are also included in this system [3].

The patients diagnosed with oral cancer early should start treatment immediately, as soon as possible, to not worsen the prognosis. At advanced stages, oral cancer (especially in stages III and IV) has a very low survival rate at 9–50% [2, 4, 14]. According to some literature, 30% of patients' efforts to seek out or find professional help for about 3 months without any intervention to malignancy but 1 month of delaying causes stage advancing and also dramatically reduces odds of survival [4, 21].

Diagnoses of oral cancer have been carried out to date by using clinical, radiological, and histopathological tools. In recent years, new technological tools and biomarkers have begun promising use as tools to diagnose oral cancer early. It can be caught in stages of cancer as early as stages I and II [10]. In addition, nanotechnology has started to see its use in diagnosing oral cancer [15]. Besides this, biomarkers were suggested to be used in detecting the malign transformation potential of premalignant lesions such as oral leukoplakia [22].

The other issue: public awareness about premalignant lesions and formed oral cancer is very important to prevent or to cure them without any morbidity or threat to life [3, 4, 8, 22]. Public awareness about self-inspection of the mouth tissue and individuals recognizing the appearance of oral cancer is crucial [3, 4]. Fortunately, in the literature, there are many actions taken on this topic [2, 8] that should be continued by healthcare providers; also, world governments should support healthcare providers' works and actions [1, 4, 8, 22] because the prognosis of oral cancer is continuing to worsen survival rates due to utilizing these pathologies at advanced stages [22].

Oral cancer has still been challenging for public health and requires significant, demanding efforts [2, 3, 7, 23, 24]. The management of oral cancer is a complex issue that requires a multidisciplinary approach, including oral and maxillofacial surgeons, oral and maxillofacial radiologists, ENT specialists, medical and radiological oncologists, prosthodontists, dentists, general surgeons, primary care clinicians (such as family medicine), physical therapy and rehabilitation specialists, dietitians, speech therapists, supportive care experts, and also pathologists or, if possible, oral and maxillofacial pathologists [2, 24, 25].

After radical, surgical, and other treatment modalities such as radiotherapy and chemotherapy—especially in stages III and IV patients—improving a patient's quality of life is very important [7, 14, 24, 26, 27]. Besides these, if patients have more advanced surgical (and other) treatment modality, the important thing is, of course, survival. Also, the second issue is improving quality of life. In this aspect, prosthodontics, speech therapy, dental implant-supported restoration with oral and maxillofacial surgeons, and other supportive specialties such as providers like physical therapists, mental health professionals, and dietitians and applications improve a patient's quality of life [2, 24].

2. Preventive awareness and control care for oral cancers

Preventive medicine acts as a unique control for oral cancers and also charges at all-time low costs to states across the world [2, 15]. In this way, many actions can be taken by health organizations, especially by the World Health Organization in the risky geographic regions of the world [28]. Prevention of oral cancer is mainly a management of those diseases, so public awareness should be the first priority for health workers (e.g., by using media to promote fast outcomes) [3, 14]. For awareness about encountering precancerous lesions [1, 22, 28], Jeihooni et al. [9] reported that 30.4% of patients had preventable oral cancer, while 50% did not, and the remaining 19.6% of patients were unclear as to whether or not oral cancer is preventable.

To prevent oral cancers, the etiological factors should be known, and measures must be taken according to those causes. Etiological factors are tobacco use, especially in individuals older than 40 years of age, alcohol consumption, betel chewing, HPV infection or carriage, dietary intakes such as salted meat consumption, poor oral hygiene, genetic predisposition, Epstein-Barr virus (EBV) infection, long-term exposure to sunlight, and immune system disease such as organ transplant recipients and HIV-infected patients, especially as it causes lip cancer [1, 3, 4, 9, 13, 14, 29, 30].

HPV-related oral cancers, especially oropharyngeal cancers, differ from other cause-related cancers as HPV-related cancers have been seen in young, non- or former tobacco users, nonalcoholic patients, and also patients with small T tumors but with nodal involvement (fortunately, their prognosis is more satisfactory than non-related HPV tumors). In addition, HPV-related tumors are well-defined borderline, more exophytic with smaller sizes and lymph node metastasis with dominant cystic features [19]. To prevent HPV-related oral cancers, vaccination against HPV should be performed to decrease the incidence of oropharyngeal SCC [31], whereas Owosho et al. [31] reported that HPV-related oropharyngeal cancer reached its highest rate in the year 2006 and has since started to decline but not at a statistically significant rate. In the literature, vaccination programs have primarily focused on HPV infection related to cervical cancer [1]. Thus, Center for Disease Control and Prevention (CDC) is recommending that the vaccination program for HPV-related oropharyngeal cancers should be carried out for children at ages 11–12 in two doses by health providers [31].

Other efforts to prevent oral cancer should be done by controlling tobacco use or reduction programs [3, 6, 7, 11, 14, 29]. Alcohol consumption should be reduced or cut off as well [3, 7, 14]. If tobacco and alcohol are used together by the same individuals, that increases the oral cancer rate and may be a dramatically worse prognosis than HPV-related cancers [3, 5, 7, 11]. Unfortunately, alcohol is related to a very risky factor for cancer occurring even in non-smoking individuals [3, 5, 7].

On the other hand, improving especially rich vegetable and fruit diet intake awareness programs, physical activity-increasing programs in daily life, regular sexual education for adolescents, and oral hygiene education activities may be helpful for reducing oral cancer rates in the future [1, 14, 32]. Awareness programs and activities should be conducted by healthcare providers or governments worldwide, especially in more risky regions such as Southeast Asia. For example, images of early oral cancer can be placed on cigarette packages [4].

In the risky region, or those patients that have high risk, they should be encouraged to carry out self-inspection of their oral mucosa, and if they see any mouth abnormality, they are obligated to take professional advice or treatment [4]. In addition, oral hygiene education and encouragement to improve it in individuals are key factors in preventing or early detection of oral cancer [9]. Moreover, Rahmati-Najarkolaei et al. [32] reported that awareness activities with students about risky factors decreased fear of oral cancer and also changed their attitude about knowing whether they have oral cancer. Lack of public awareness about cancer-causing factors and predictors produces diagnosis of oral cancer at stages as late as III or IV [4]. Therefore, awareness may provide early diagnosing of lesions; it reduces the cost of treatment and also reduces treatment morbidity [16, 22].

To date, many strategies have experimented with community awareness in the literature, such as mass media campaigns, which have gained some success from increased public awareness [1, 3, 8]. Unfortunately, these improvements are still not enough in terms of public awareness. Nowadays, Internet-based or online connections such as social media are very popular communication tools across the whole world. For example, the online-supported education or activities for tobacco cessation counseling revealed limited success in a randomized experiment [1, 8]. Internet-based education also applied for alcohol counseling with some success gained [1]. Billboards have also not been successful in delivering improved awareness to risky populations [1]. Prevention is the main management of oral cancers, and public awareness is a key part of prevention: where, when, and how it should be done and how it is possible is not important.

2.1. Look and see: precancerous mouth lesions

Many types of oral lesions have malignant transformation potential, aptly named premalignant or precancerous lesions. Premalignant lesions are described by using clinical, pathological, histochemical, and also many other screening techniques for which lesions such as leukoplakia, lichen planus with oral and cutaneous form, erythroplakia, stomatitis nicotina, and submucous fibrosis are named or classified [3, 10, 15, 18, 22, 33–35]. In addition, there is less malign transformation potential in lesions such as discoid lupus erythematosus and also a lesser likelihood of malignant transformation in hereditary entities such as epidermolysis bullosa and dyskeratosis congenita [34]. For the lip cancer, there are precancerous lesions like xeroderma pigmentosum, radiodermatitis, and chronic cheilitis [18]. However, histological investigation has only produced knowledge about malignant transformation potential—named dysplasia—and has been indicated or used as a prediction of malignant changes [34]. According to the WHO's (2005) statement, carcinoma in situ has the highest degree of dysplasia and is also defined as a premalignant lesion [3, 10, 34]. Premalignant lesions are usually clinically screened for mouth mucosa such as white, red, or red-white mixed patches and are also called leukoplakia or erythroplakia [34, 35].

3. Early diagnosis of precancerous and oral cancer lesion techniques

Early detection of premalignant lesions and also cancer lesions is a crucial issue for the head and neck region, as the late diagnosing rate of 60% worldwide causes huge surgical and oncological interventions or low survival rate [14, 15, 36]. To date, there are many clinical, histopathological, radiological, and optical techniques to diagnose or capture precancerous and oral cancer lesions, such as vital tissue staining (toluidine blue stain), exfoliative cytology, OralCDx (OralCDx Laboratories, Suffern, NY) or Orcellex® (Rovers Medical Devices, BV, the Netherlands), brush cytology, and cell markers or biomarkers. There are also many new developments of novel real-time in vivo imaging and spectroscopy-based devices: high-resolution microendoscopy (HRME), autofluorescence imaging (AFI), targeted fluorescence imaging (TFI), and optical coherence tomography (OCT); also, there are other optical visualization methods such as ViziLite Plus with Orascoptic DK (Orascoptic, a Kerr Company, Middleton, Wis.), VELscope™ (Visually Enhanced Lesion Scope, LED Dental, White Rock, British Columbia, Canada), Microlux DL (AdDent, Danbury, Conn.), ViziLite (Zila Pharmaceuticals), TBlue (Zila Pharmaceuticals, Phoenix), Raman spectroscopy (RS), elastic scattering spectroscopy (ESS), narrowband imaging (NBI), diffuse reflectance spectroscopy (DRS), and confocal reflectance microscopy (CRM) in addition to normal biopsy of the tissue with histopathological investigation [12, 15, 16, 28, 34–38].

These techniques are local detectors of lesions. Besides these, oral cancer may spread regionally and may also have distant metastasis. For instance, to make stage determining and treatment strategies for lesions, imaging systems as computed tomography (CT), magnetic resonance imaging (MRI), cone beam computerized tomography (CBCT), and positron emission tomography (PET) can be useful to scan the head and neck region for regional spread of oral cancer [15]. These techniques are divided into two categories, as either lesion detection or lesion assessment. Whether these tests have been tested across several works, however, remains questionable [37].

Toluidine blue stain is a metachromatic thiazine material that binds to DNA in alcohol and water. Toluidine blue (TB) is a member of the thiazine group of metachromatic dyes, which binds to DNA and is partially soluble both in water and in alcohol. Theoretically, dysplastic and malignant cells have higher nucleic acid content; hence, it is stained with dyes that can be identified under the microscope due to nucleic acid and have been used since 1980 [34]. Toluidine blue stain, ViziLite, and VEL scope sensitivity and specificity in oral dysplasia patients are presented by Awan et al. [37] to be 84.1 and 77.3%, 15.3 and 27.8%, and 65.8 and 56.8%, respectively.

Exfoliative cytology procures cells from a wide surface area of the affected tissue with fewer invasive effects on the tissue than biopsy. It also involves a lower contamination risk prior to DNA obtaining than surgical intervention [5]. Exfoliative cytology is obtained by scrapping the mucosa lesion using a blade as tongue blade. The obtained material is spread on a dry, clean glass lam and fixed with 100% ethanol. The lam is then sent to an experienced pathologist for examination under a light microscope for dysplastic evidences in the cells [35]. In addition, serum and saliva are the most commonly used as less invasive, easily accessible, cost-effective, and convenient samples for cancer detection [15]. The sensitivity and specificity of exfoliative cytology for oral cancer detection were revealed as 93.5 and 50.6%, respectively [15]. Although exfoliative cytology is less invasive, it is highly subjective and dependent upon the expertise of examiners. Moreover, exfoliative cytology related to the DNA aneuploidy and quantitative cytomorphometry has low specificity due to the collection of disassembled cells [15]. If the exfoliative cytology is used on heavy smoker and alcohol-using patients with negative malignancy findings, a biopsy procedure should be carried out as an additional supportive test [22].

OralCDx or Orcellex® brush cytology is a bit advanced for complementary forms of the exfoliative cytology, due to it including representative cells of all layers of epithelial tissue [34, 38]. Moreover, brush cytology has provided diagnostic accuracy because of computer assistance screening [34, 38]. Studies demonstrated that OralCDx or Orcellex® cytology has a potential value as an adjunct to oral diagnosing or screening in identifying premalignant pathologies at early stages that provides surgical or curative treatment that is most effective [39]. In the future, developing automatic, cytometric, or cytomorphometric techniques combined with genetic and related features may enhance screening strategies [34]. Affecting tissue with any pathology sample technique is still recommended if there is a strong suspicion of any lesion with malignancy regardless of the oral brush cytology result [34].

Biological, chemical, or reactional molecular agents named cell markers and biomarkers mean that signs of living organisms and the obviousness of their availability as tumor necrosis factor-alpha (TNF-α), epithelial growth factor (EGFR), vascular endothelial growth factor (VEGF), IL-8 and IL-8 mRNA, and interleukin 6 (IL-6) [10, 15]. Biomarker investigation of abnormalities of oral tissues as normal, tumorous, and inflammatory keratinocyte proteomes is likely to find new biomarker agents for oral cancer diagnosis, treatment, follow-up, and the development of personalized therapies for oral cancer and other tumorous regions [16].

The most visible oral premalignant or precancerous lesion is oral leukoplakia (OL) that has been studied for its establishment of a biomarker that signals the malign transformation of OL [22]. For instance, OL has low prevalence in western countries, so the development of a new biomarker is challenging due to the low rate of malignant transformation, and it requires long follow-up periods to achieve a new biomarker [22]. Besides these, loss of heterozygosity (LOH) was described as the strongest and most valuable biomarker by Mao et al. at the end of the twentieth century. They reported that OL housing LOH at 3p14 or 9p21 was related to the 37% chance of developing invasive cancer compared with only 6% in lesions without these biomarkers [22]. Dysplasia is a very important sign of OL malign transformation; however, it does not mean that it will transform into a malign lesion, such as an oral squamous cell carcinoma lesion. Detecting or signaling oral leukoplakia malignant-transforming biomarkers is crucial in the future. Chemoprevention actions or works using retinoid evoked unique prospective gathering of biodata that led to the development of biomarkers [22]. Evidence-based studies showed that a visual examination of oral regions may be a cost-effective screening model, and finding adjunct auxiliaries and biomarkers is becoming more popular [28].

Hence, if the environmental conditions could be changed, oral leukoplakia may be reversible even with advanced dysplasia, which does not change into any malign lesion such as OSCC [22]. However, the existence of dysplasia is often the important criterion that affects clinical treatment of oral leukoplakia [22].

Microendoscopy (HRME) is a novel in vivo optical imaging and spectroscopy-based tool that has the content to provide an early diagnosis of cancer in real time. This tool is a cost-effective and noninvasive technique for point-of-care detection of premalignant and cancer in body regions including the oral cavity and hypopharynx. The HRME technique provides direct screening of malignant indicators such as nuclear crowding, pleomorphism, and elevated nuclear-to-cytoplasmic area ratio. This technique has almost identical possibility with cytology and invasive biopsy procedures. The HRME technique therefore has a promising development in the future [36, 40].

The ViziLite system, as an oral optical lumenoscopy technique alone or in combination with other techniques mentioned above, has been used successfully in the last decade. The US Food and Drug Administration has received a combination of both ViziLite and TB systems (ViziLite Plus with TBlue System; Zila, Batesville, AR, USA), as an adjunct to visual screening of the oral cavity. This combined technique for detecting or diagnosing premalignant or cancerous lesions provides almost the same level of outcome that invasive method biopsy and histopathological investigation provide [15, 22, 34, 37].

VELscope™ (LED Dental, White Rock, British Columbia, Canada) is noninvasive and directly screens the changes of tissue autofluorescence characteristic screening tools in the oral cavity [12, 22]. It uses blue light between 400 and 460 nm wavelengths to influence the endogenous fluorophores. Because of its simplicity, it does not require any special training on the system and can be used in daily general subspecialty practice. Farah et al. [41] reported that VELscope™ screening did not provide a definitive diagnosis on the existence of epithelial dysplasia, so VELscope™ is not reliable for detecting epithelial dysplasia without clinical examination. In contrast to the Farah et al. [41] report, the other study carried out by Awan et al. [42] reported that VELscope™ is useful in confirming the existence of erythroplakia, oral leukoplakia, and other soft tissue diseases, but it cannot discriminate between low-risk and high-risk pathologies [34].

Raman spectroscopy (RS), a common optical diagnostic technique, works with vibrational spectroscopies that discriminate normal mucosa and malignant pathologies by reflecting variables within tissues and returning optical signals [15]. However, this optical tool's original yet

http://dx.doi.org/10.5772/intechopen.81126

subjective finding outcomes depend on the practitioners' evaluation experience [15]. Stone et al. [43] first applied the Raman spectroscopy in the head and neck region in 2000 to investigate the laryngeal mucosa by comparing with normal biopsy procedures in 15 patients. According to this study, RS produced a specificity of 90 and 92% sensitivity for detecting squamous cell carcinoma [43]. We may thus conclude that the RS technique is useful for daily practice.

3.1. Multidisciplinary approach to diagnosis and management of precancerous and oral cancer lesions: healthcare providers and patients' role

Early diagnosis, a crucial issue as mentioned above, is very easy, but across the world, oral cancer is being detected in late stage due to its subtlety in early stage [3]. The routine management of oral cancer is first surgical resection, with or without postoperative adjuncts and other therapies used as part of postoperative chemoradiation and radiation. This approach of combining multiple treatments has increased survival rates in the last decade.

Successful treatment of oral cancer patients is a complex issue that requires multidisciplinary approaches, including oral and maxillofacial surgeons, oral and maxillofacial radiologists, ENT specialists, medical and radiological oncologists, prosthodontists, dentists, general surgeons, primary care clinicians (such as family medicine), physical therapy and rehabilitation specialists, dietitians, speech therapists, supportive care experts, and also pathologists or, if possible, oral and maxillofacial pathologists [2, 3, 24, 25]. In addition, multidisciplinary approaches to oral cancer patients allow for the maximization of reliable oncologic control and also minimize morbidities such as patient function and form [3].

Early diagnosis of oral cancer is vital for a patient's survival rate and also for future quality of life. In addition, a dentist has an important role in initial diagnosing of any pathology in the oral region because of daily oral health practice [2, 14, 43]. So, any ignorance on behalf of dentists' education and daily practice is a crucial phenomenon for detecting any lesions in early phase. If a dentist has detected any abnormality of oral tissue in an emergency situation, he or she should perform a biopsy procedure or immediately refer the patients to advanced specialties such as oral and maxillofacial surgeons, otolaryngologists, or advanced oncological-trained oral and maxillofacial surgeons, if it is possible [2, 14].

In a majority of world regions, the oral and maxillofacial surgery specialty is based on dentistry education and is concerned with diagnosis, medical and surgical, and advanced treatment of disease, disorders, injuries, and malformation, including the functional and esthetic features of the oral and maxillofacial region's soft and hard tissues and related neighboring structures [2]. Oral and maxillofacial surgeons take part in the biopsy, which checks whether it is a true- or false-positive diagnosis; advanced radiological imaging is required to investigate in this stage of pathology. In addition, they surgically treat precancerous lesions and also take part in the treatment of early-stage cancer.

A case with a 67-year-old male patient was referred to an experienced oral and maxillofacial surgeon and diagnosed with oral leukoplakia. The patient was treated with a diode laser using evaporation mode. According to the follow-up period, no recurrence has been revealed with the patient in healthy oral condition (**Figures 1** and **2**).

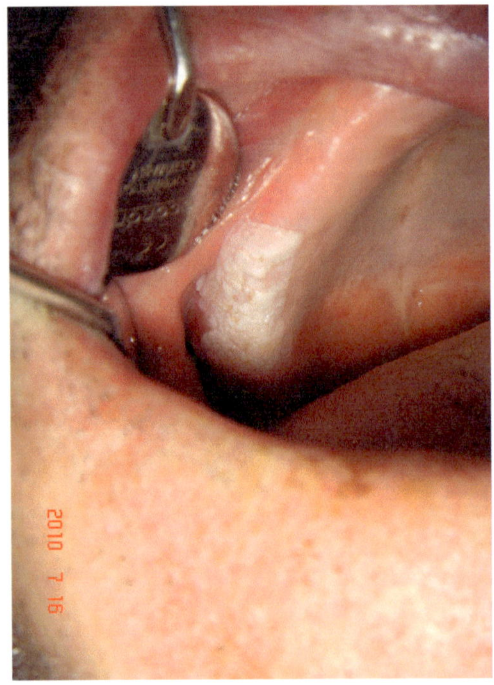

Figure 1 . Prelaser treatment of oral leukoplakia (Case 1 patient).

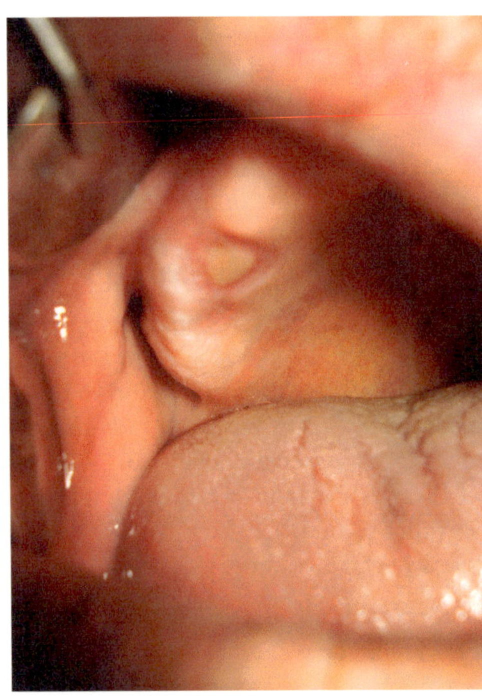

Figure 2 . Postoperative laser treatment view of oral leukoplakia (Case 1 patient).

If the OMF surgeon has not accrued enough experience for more extensive pathology, he or she should refer patients to trained or sufficiently experienced head and neck surgeons such as an oral and maxillofacial surgeon, ear nose throat surgeon, general surgeon, or a plastic surgeon; plastic surgeons and oral and maxillofacial surgeons have a duty to perform pre-prosthetic surgery, revision surgery, and also dental and oral and maxillofacial implants to rehabilitate the oral cavity for speech improvement, swallowing, mastication, and esthetic appearance. In addition, oral and maxillofacial surgeons promote maxillofacial prosthodontists for the construction of maxillofacial and oral prosthesis [2].

Oral and maxillofacial oncology training was part of a related oral and maxillofacial surgery residency program for about 3–4 years, following the 5–6 years for a basic dentistry degree. In addition, these specially trained people take an additional 1 or 2 years' oncological surgery training for cancer surgery and rehabilitation and reconstruction surgery such as regional vascular flap reconstruction, e.g., a pectoralis major flap with five to six costal grafts, a latissimus dorsi muscular flap with scapular graft, and other regional soft and hard tissue vascular flaps to reconstruct mandibular and maxillary resection defects are used. In addition, distant vascular-free flaps such as perineal musculocutaneous with fibula and an anterior radial forearm flap are used to reconstruct maxillary and mandibular oncologic resected defects by oral and maxillofacial oncologic program surgeons. On the other hand, the oncologic oral and maxillofacial surgeon training program includes core rotations on resection and reconstruction surgery, medical oncology, and radiation oncology. They also carry out duties like educating others in the dental profession on cancer screening and management. They take part in the oncological multidisciplinary team, including pathologists, radiologists, ENT specialists, and other professions [2].

The transoral access is a common surgical approach to precancerous pathologies and superficial cancers of anterior portions of the mouth, tongue, and alveolus. In the posterior region of the mouth, an invasive approach is needed, especially if there is a limitation due to inadequate surgical view and trismus. Median lip-split paramedian mandibulotomy access is used for tumor management of the posterior mouth region. In addition, midfacial degloving and upper cheek access are typically useful for maxillary tumors [3].

Neck dissection is a very important part of oral cancer surgical management. Fortunately, 60% of cases with an early-stage tumor have clinically negative neck metastasis. Unfortunately, nearly 20–30% of entities have microscopically prominent neck nodal metastasis according to elective neck dissection (END). Nodal metastasis risk occurs for several reasons. One, cervical lymph node metastasis can reduce the survival rate by 50% when compared with similar primary tumors, excepting cervical or other regions. Tongue cancer on the mouth floor is more likely to advance into the neck lymph node; thus, these cases should require elective neck dissection, even if they are in an early stage.

The maxillary gum and hard palate have relatively lower chances of neck metastasis occurring, and if this is determined to be the case, there is no need for END to be indicated [3].

Isolated node biopsy is an adjunct alternative to END for determining the stage of a cN0 neck in the T1–T2 stage of SCCOC [3, 44]. This method was first carried out in 2001 by Shoaib et al. [44], and it has been used by several other studies in Europe and the USA. However, this

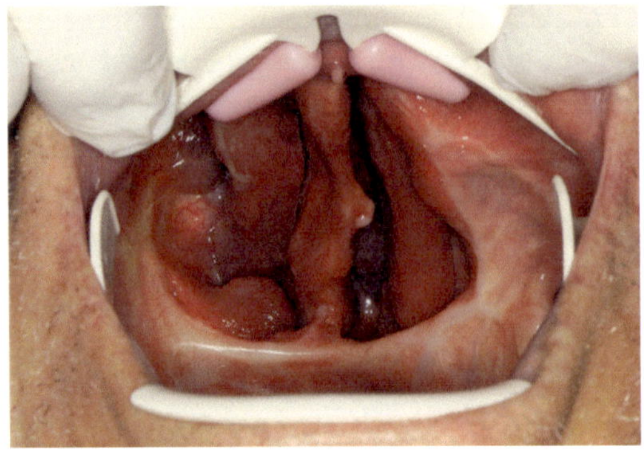

Figure 3 . Prereconstruction dentures' view of Case 2 patient's oral structures after a maxillary cancer operation.

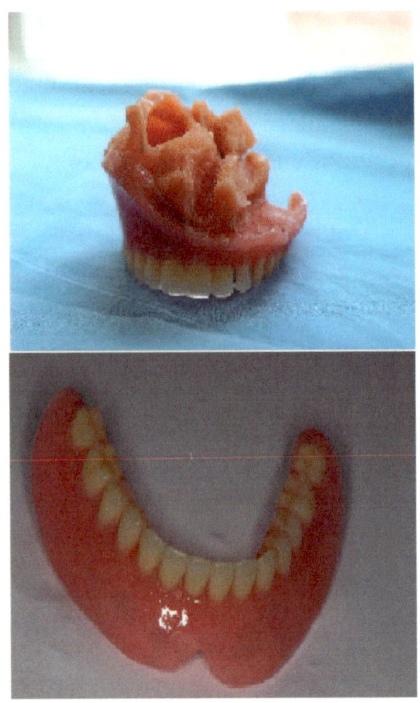

Figure 4 . Maxillomandibular dentures' view of Case 2 patient.

technique requires experienced practitioners to be able to carry out the procedure. It should therefore be done in select centers with experienced doctors [3].

If patients are clinically or radiographically determined to have positive neck nodes, a comprehensive neck dissection should be done involving level I to V dissection. The requirement to sacrifice important structures like the sternocleidomastoid muscle, spinal accessory nerve, and internal jugular vein depends on the location of the nodal metastasis and its features [44]. A common type of wide neck dissection is the modified radical neck dissection, named MRND type 1. MRND, as a treatment choice, is a rarely selected option due to direct infiltration of

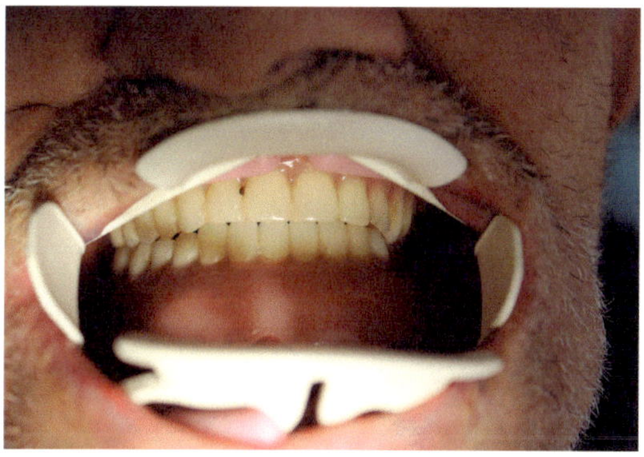

Figure 5 . The appearance of prosthetic dentures placed in Case 2 patient.

the gross extranodal structures [3]. A patient with clinically negative neck node metastasis has metastasis risk mainly throughout levels I to III. Therefore, supraomohyoid neck dissection (SOHND) is usually enough for these diseases. However, patients with primary tongue squamous cell carcinoma require neck dissection level IV and may be obligated due to the likelihood of skip metastasis [3].

Oral pathologists and oral medicine specialists also play key roles in oral cancer prevention, diagnosing, early management, and follow-up procedures. They perform the biopsy procedures in oral pathologies that identify lesions; hence, strategies are formed for the management process of the detected lesion [2].

Maxillofacial prosthodontists take part in key positions in management specifically to restore the function of jaws and maxillofacial tissue after tumor eradication. To improve the patients' psychological condition, they replace the functional and cosmetic defects with prosthetic construction carried out by prosthodontics in the maxillofacial region [2].

Case 2 features a 78-year-old male patient who underwent total maxillectomy due to squamous cell carcinoma. With an oral and maxillofacial surgeon's guidance, to improve the life quality of the patient, the maxillomandibular dentures were constructed by an experienced prosthodontist. The patient is chewing and eating smoothly, and he is still under the control period in uneventful condition (**Figures 3–5**).

Acknowledgements

The authors of this chapter thank IntechOpen for providing a unique opportunity to contribute to the book *Oral Cancer*.

Conflict of interest

The authors of this manuscript declare that they have no conflict of interest.

Author details

Nihat Akbulut* and Ahmet Altan

*Address all correspondence to: drnihatakbulut@yahoo.com

Oral and Maxillofacial Surgery Department, Faculty of Dentistry, Tokat Gaziosmanpasa University, Tokat, Turkey

References

[1] LeHew CW, Weatherspoon DJ, Peterson CE, Goben A, Reitmajer K, Sroussi H, et al. The health system and policy implications of changing epidemiology for oral cavity and oropharyngeal cancers in the United States from 1995 to 2016. Epidemiologic Reviews. 2017;**39**(1):132-147

[2] Yadav SK. Oral cancer care and oromaxillofacial surgery. Journal of Nepal Health Research Council. 2015;**13**(30):169-174

[3] Montero PH, Patel SG. Cancer of the oral cavity. Surgical Oncology Clinics of North America. 2015;**24**(3):491-508

[4] Hassona Y, Sawair F, Matarweh D, Abdalhamid A, Thweib D, Scully C. Oral cancer early detection: What do patients need to know? Journal of Cancer Education. Aug 2018;**33**(4):865-869

[5] Termine N, Giovannelli L, Rodolico V, Matranga D, Pannone G, Campisi G. Biopsy vs. brushing: Comparison of two sampling methods for the detection of HPV-DNA in squamous cell carcinoma of the oral cavity. Oral Oncology. 2012;**48**(9):870-875

[6] Ang KK, Harris J, Wheeler R, Weber R, Rosenthal DI, Nguyen-Tan PF, et al. Human papillomavirus and survival of patients with oropharyngeal cancer. The New England Journal of Medicine. 2010;**363**(1):24-35

[7] D'Cruz A, Lin T, Anand AK, Atmakusuma D, Calaguas MJ, Chitapanarux I, et al. Consensus recommendations for management of head and neck cancer in Asian countries: A review of international guidelines. Oral Oncology. 2013;**49**(9):872-877

[8] Saleh A, Yang YH, Wan Abd Ghani WM, Abdullah N, Doss JG, Navonil R, et al. Promoting oral cancer awareness and early detection using a mass media approach. Asian Pacific Journal of Cancer Prevention: APJCP. 2012;**13**(4):1217-1224

[9] Jeihooni AK, Dindarloo SF, Harsini PA. Effectiveness of health belief model on oral cancer prevention in smoker men. Journal of Cancer Education. Jul 11 2018. DOI: 10.1007/s13187-018-1396-7 [Epub ahead of print]

[10] Chang YA, Weng SL, Yang SF, Chou CH, Huang WC, Tu SJ, et al. A three-microRNA signature as a potential biomarker for the early detection of oral cancer. International Journal of Molecular Sciences. Mar 7 2018;**19**(3). DOI: 10.3390/ijms19030758 [Epub ahead of print]

[11] Blatt S, Ziebart T, Kruger M, Pabst AM. Diagnosing oral squamous cell carcinoma: How much imaging do we really need? A review of the current literature. Journal of Cranio-Maxillo-Facial Surgery: Official Publication of the European Association for Cranio-Maxillo-Facial Surgery. 2016;**44**(5):538-549

[12] Wu C, Gleysteen J, Teraphongphom NT, Li Y, Rosenthal E. In-vivo optical imaging in head and neck oncology: Basic principles, clinical applications and future directions. International Journal of Oral Science. 2018;**10**(2):10

[13] Arya S, Rane P, Deshmukh A. Oral cavity squamous cell carcinoma: Role of pretreatment imaging and its influence on management. Clinical Radiology. 2014;**69**(9):916-930

[14] Akbulut N, Oztas B, Kursun S, Evirgen S. Delayed diagnosis of oral squamous cell carcinoma: A case series. Journal of Medical Case Reports. 2011;**5**:291

[15] Chen XJ, Zhang XQ, Liu Q, Zhang J, Zhou G. Nanotechnology: A promising method for oral cancer detection and diagnosis. Journal of Nanobiotechnology. 2018;**16**(1):52

[16] Lupu M, Caruntu A, Caruntu C, Boda D, Moraru L, Voiculescu V, et al. Non-invasive imaging of actinic cheilitis and squamous cell carcinoma of the lip. Molecular and Clinical Oncology. 2018;**8**(5):640-646

[17] Chan KK, Glenny AM, Weldon JC, Furness S, Worthington HV, Wakeford H. Interventions for the treatment of oral and oropharyngeal cancers: Targeted therapy and immunotherapy. The Cochrane Database of Systematic Reviews. 2015;**12**:CD010341

[18] Vukadinovic M, Jezdic Z, Petrovic M, Medenica LM, Lens M. Surgical management of squamous cell carcinoma of the lip: Analysis of a 10 year experience in 223 patients. Journal of Oral and Maxillofacial Surgery: Official Journal of the American Association of Oral and Maxillofacial Surgeons. 2007;**65**(4):675-679

[19] Denaro N, Russi EG, Merlano MC. Pros and cons of the new edition of TNM classification of head and neck squamous cell carcinoma. Oncology. 2018;**95**(4):202-210

[20] Bezerra NV, Leite KL, de Medeiros MM, Martins ML, Cardoso AM, Alves PM, et al. Impact of the anatomical location, alcoholism and smoking on the prevalence of advanced oral cancer in Brazil. Medicina Oral, Patología Oral y Cirugía Bucal. 2018;**23**(3):e295-e301

[21] Dantas TS, de Barros Silva PG, Sousa EF, da Cunha Mdo P, de Aguiar AS, Costa FW, et al. Influence of educational level, stage, and histological type on survival of oral cancer in a Brazilian population: A retrospective study of 10 years observation. Medicine. 2016;**95**(3):e2314

[22] Foy JP, Bertolus C, William WN Jr, Saintigny P. Oral premalignancy: The roles of early detection and chemoprevention. Otolaryngologic Clinics of North America. 2013;**46**(4):579-597

[23] Shah JP, Gil Z. Current concepts in management of oral cancer-surgery. Oral Oncology. 2009;**45**(4-5):394-401

[24] Nekhlyudov L, Lacchetti C, Davis NB, Garvey TQ, Goldstein DP, Nunnink JC, et al. Head and neck cancer survivorship care guideline: American Society of Clinical Oncology

clinical practice guideline endorsement of the American Cancer Society guideline. Journal of Clinical Oncology: Official Journal of the American Society of Clinical Oncology. 2017;**35**(14):1606-1621

[25] Dougherty W, Givi B, Jameson MJ, Education Committee of the American H, Neck S. AHNS series—Do you know your guidelines? Lip cancer. Head & Neck. 2017; **39**(8):1505-1509

[26] Mucke T, Koschinski J, Wolff KD, Kanatas A, Mitchell DA, Loeffelbein DJ, et al. Quality of life after different oncologic interventions in head and neck cancer patients. Journal of Cranio-Maxillo-Facial Surgery: Official Publication of the European Association for Cranio-Maxillo-Facial Surgery. 2015;**43**(9):1895-1898

[27] Rogers SN. Quality of life for head and neck cancer patients-has treatment planning altered? Oral Oncology. 2009;**45**(4-5):435-439

[28] Brocklehurst P, Kujan O, O'Malley LA, Ogden G, Shepherd S, Glenny AM. Screening programmes for the early detection and prevention of oral cancer. The Cochrane Database of Systematic Reviews. 2013;**11**:CD004150

[29] Priya M, Lando HA. Tobacco control: An issue twinned with oral cancer control. International Dental Journal. 2014;**64**(5):229-232

[30] Maggioni D, Biffi L, Nicolini G, Garavello W. Flavonoids in oral cancer prevention and therapy. European Journal of Cancer Prevention: The Official Journal of the European Cancer Prevention Organisation. 2015;**24**(6):517-528

[31] Owosho AA, Wiley R, Stansbury T, Gbadamosi SO, Ryder JS. Trends in human papillomavirus-related oropharyngeal squamous cell carcinoma incidence, Vermont 1999-2013. Journal of Community Health. 2018;**43**(4):731-737

[32] Rahmati-Najarkolaei F, Rahnama P, Gholami Fesharaki M, Behnood V. Predictors of oral health behaviors in female students: An application of the health belief model. Iranian Red Crescent Medical Journal. 2016;**18**(11):e24747

[33] Wang KH, Song BH, Gilde JE, Darbinian JA, Weintraub MLR, Wu TJ, et al. Diagnostic pathway of oral cavity cancer in an integrated health care system. The Permanente Journal. Mar 30 2018;22. DOI: 10.7812/TPP/17-152

[34] Messadi DV. Diagnostic aids for detection of oral precancerous conditions. International Journal of Oral Science. 2013;**5**(2):59-65

[35] Gupta S, Shah JS, Parikh S, Limbdiwala P, Goel S. Clinical correlative study on early detection of oral cancer and precancerous lesions by modified oral brush biopsy and cytology followed by histopathology. Journal of Cancer Research and Therapeutics. 2014;**10**(2):232-238

[36] Guze K, Pawluk HC, Short M, Zeng H, Lorch J, Norris C, et al. Pilot study: Raman spectroscopy in differentiating premalignant and malignant oral lesions from normal mucosa and benign lesions in humans. Head & Neck. 2015;**37**(4):511-517

[37] Awan KH, Morgan PR, Warnakulasuriya S. Assessing the accuracy of autofluorescence, chemiluminescence and toluidine blue as diagnostic tools for oral potentially malignant disorders—A clinicopathological evaluation. Clinical Oral Investigations. 2015;**19**(9):2267-2272

[38] Alsarraf A, Kujan O, Farah CS. Liquid-based oral brush cytology in the diagnosis of oral leukoplakia using a modified Bethesda cytology system. Journal of Oral Pathology & Medicine. Jun 29 2018. DOI: 10.1111/jop.12759 [Epub ahead of print]

[39] Sciubba JJ. Improving detection of precancerous and cancerous oral lesions. Computer-assisted analysis of the oral brush biopsy. U. S. collaborative OralCDx study group. Journal of the American Dental Association. 1999;**130**(10):1445-1457

[40] Ishijima A, Schwarz RA, Shin D, Mondrik S, Vigneswaran N, Gillenwater AM, et al. Automated frame selection process for high-resolution microendoscopy. Journal of Biomedical Optics. 2015;**20**(4):46014

[41] Farah CS, McIntosh L, Georgiou A, McCullough MJ. Efficacy of tissue autofluorescence imaging (VELScope) in the visualization of oral mucosal lesions. Head & Neck. 2012;**34**(6):856-862

[42] Awan KH, Morgan PR, Warnakulasuriya S. Evaluation of an autofluorescence based imaging system (VELscope) in the detection of oral potentially malignant disorders and benign keratoses. Oral Oncology. 2011;**47**(4):274-277

[43] Stone N, Stavroulaki P, Kendall C, Birchall M, Barr H. Raman spectroscopy for early detection of laryngeal malignancy: Preliminary results. The Laryngoscope. 2000;**110**(10 Pt 1):1756-1763

[44] Shoaib T, Soutar DS, MacDonald DG, Camilleri IG, Dunaway DJ, Gray HW, et al. The accuracy of head and neck carcinoma sentinel lymph node biopsy in the clinically N0 neck. Cancer. 2001;**91**(11):2077-2083

Chapter 5

Management Strategies for Oral Cancer Subsites

Neeti Kapre Gupta, Monica Mahajan and
Apeksha Hore

Additional information is available at the end of the chapter

http://dx.doi.org/10.5772/intechopen.81555

Abstract

Oral cancers are the most common cancers in India, especially in males. This can be attributed primarily to consumption of tobacco and areca related products. Surgery is the mainstay of treatment for oral cancers with subtle subsite-specific nuances. The oral cavity starts at the mucocutaneous junction of the lips (the vermilion border) extending posteriorly to the junction of the hard and soft palate superiorly, anterior fauces laterally and the junction of the anterior two-thirds and posterior third of the tongue inferiorly. The oral cavity is lined by stratified squamous epithelium of varying degrees of keratinization. Primary tumors of the oral cavity may be derived from the mucosa, salivary glands, neurovascular tissues, bone or dental tissues. Over 90% of malignant tumors of the oral cavity are squamous cell carcinomas. There are certain basic principles of oncology, those hold true, despite the disease subsite and pathology. Stage I and II disease should be dealt with single modality treatment, whereas Stage III and IV warrant combined modality approach. Choice of modality (surgical versus non-surgical), depends on intent of treatment, chances of cure, accessibility and resectability of disease, impact on quality of life and patient's general health profile.

Keywords: oral cancer, oral oncosurgery, radiotherapy, chemotherapy

1. Introduction

Oral cancers are the most common cancers in India, especially in males. This can be attributed primarily to consumption of tobacco and areca related products. Surgery is the mainstay of treatment for oral cancers with subtle subsite-specific nuances.

The oral cavity starts at the mucocutaneous junction of the lips (the vermilion border) extending posteriorly to the junction of the hard and soft palate superiorly, anterior fauces laterally and the junction of the anterior two-thirds and posterior third of the tongue inferiorly. The oral cavity is lined by stratified squamous epithelium of varying degrees of keratinization. Primary tumors of the oral cavity may be derived from the mucosa, salivary glands, neuro-vascular tissues, bone or dental tissues. Over 90% of malignant tumors of the oral cavity are squamous cell carcinomas.

There are certain basic principles of oncology, those hold true, despite the disease subsite and pathology. Stage I and II disease should be dealt with single modality treatment, whereas Stage III and IV warrant combined modality approach. Choice of modality (surgical versus non-surgical), depends on intent of treatment, chances of cure, accessibility and resectability of disease, impact on quality of life and patient's general health profile.

The following chapter attempts to succinctly highlight subtle differences in management of oral cancer at individual subsites.

1.1. Diagnosis: imaging

Contrast enhanced multi-detector computed tomography (CECT) scan is the workhorse for head and neck imaging. Magnetic resonance imaging (MRI) is preferred for better soft tissue delineation. **Table 1** summarizes preferred imaging modality in individual subsite.

A distant metastatic work-up is indicated in oral cancers in the following scenarios-

- Patients presenting with obvious symptoms pointing to distant metastatic sites
- Recurrent disease, especially with short disease-free interval
- Extensive nodal burden/lower level (root of the neck) cervical nodes
- Primary resection is expected to be excessively morbid

Whole body contrast enhanced PETCT is the investigation of choice for these patients since it offers the combined advantage of functional and structural imaging.

Sr. no.	Site	Imaging modalities
1	Lip, buccal mucosa, gingivobuccal sulcus, mandible, retromolar trigone	Primarily: CECT (a puffed cheek technique is preferred)
2	Tongue, floor of the mouth	Primarily: MRI Other preferred modalities: CECT (especially if mandibular bone involvement is suspected)
3	Maxilla	Primarily: CT Other preferred modalities: MRI (helpful for detection of perineural invasion)
4	Hard palate	Primarily: CT Other preferred modalities: MRI

Table 1. Choice of imaging modality for individual subsites in oral cavity.

http://dx.doi.org/10.5772/intechopen.81555

1.2. Diagnosis: pathology

Biopsy and subsequent histological examination is the gold standard for diagnosing head and neck malignancies. The most representative part of the lesion should be chosen for taking punch biopsies. It is certainly not necessary to take biopsy from margin of diseased and normal tissue as was previously advocated. Verrucous proliferative lesions may harbor foci of invasive cancer in 20% cases, therefore it is essential to include reasonable depth of tissue while performing biopsy. A wedge incision or knife biopsy is often recommended in these situations. Fine needle aspiration cytology (FNAC) aids for ascertaining positive nodal metastases. Sometimes imaging guided biopsy or FNAC are useful for targeting disease in difficult to access areas. Certain specific viral antibodies testing (human papilloma virus (HPV) for oropharynx) may be supplemented as deemed necessary.

2. Treatment

Definitive treatment modalities: The management for cancer mainly includes three treatment modalities—surgery, radiotherapy and chemotherapy. These modalities can be used individually or in combination with each other. The factors that influence choice of initial treatment for primary carcinomas of the oral cavity are dependent on the characteristics of the primary tumor (tumor factors), those related to the patient—site of the primary tumor, size (T-stage), location (anterior vs. posterior), proximity to bone (mandible or maxilla), status of cervical lymph nodes, histology (type, grade, and depth of invasion), and previous treatment, and those related to the treatment team providing care to the patient (physician factors). The ultimate goals in treatment of cancer of the oral cavity are to eradicate the cancer, preserve or restore form and function, minimize the sequelae of treatment, and prevent subsequent new primary tumors [1].

2.1. Surgery

Surgery is the mainstay of treatment for oral cancers. The goal of any oncological surgery is complete removal of the primary tumor and appropriate clearance of regional lymph nodes, while preserving the integrity of uninvolved structures.

2.1.1. Management of primary lesion

The surgical plan should involve wide excision of the tumor in all three dimensions with adequate margins (**Table 2**). This should account for histopathological shrinkage (approximately 25%) [2]. Due attention must be given specially to the third dimension which is the soft tissue/depth and generally the site of surgical failures. An examination under anesthesia should ideally always precede the excision.

Intraoperative frozen section evaluation is a very effective modality to assess the complete removal of the malignant lesion. Frozen section provides instant pathological information that can guide intra-operative surgical decision making such as adequacy of margins, identification of nodal metastases [3, 4]. However, we have literature from high volume centers

Negative margin	>5 mm
Close margin	1–5 mm
Positive margin	<1 mm/tumor cut through

Table 2. Adequacy of margins for resection of oral primary.

in India to suggest that the incremental value of frozen section analysis of margins over surgeon's gross assessment is limited when the margin is >7 mm [5]. The authors have original research work in role of crush imprint cytology for identification of nodal metastases from oral cancers with reasonable sensitivity (92%) and accuracy (88%) [6].

2.1.1.1. Approaches to the oral cavity

Per-oral: This approach has the following prerequisites (**Figure 1**)

1. Adequate mouth opening
2. Small size
3. Anteriorly located lesions
4. All resection margins accessible
5. Noncontiguous lymph nodal spread

Upper cheek flap: This approach allows access to the maxilla, upper alveolus, hard palate. Care should be exercised while raising the flap superolaterally to avoid injury to the infra-orbital nerve and to anticipate subcutaneous/cutaneous soft tissue extent of the tumor while deciding the thickness of the flap. Extensions of the flap such as the lateral rhinotomy, Weber Ferguson with or without Dieffenbach extension can be used to excise sinonasal tumors. Lateral subciliary or supra-orbital incisions can be combined to perform orbital exenteration depending upon the extent of the tumor.

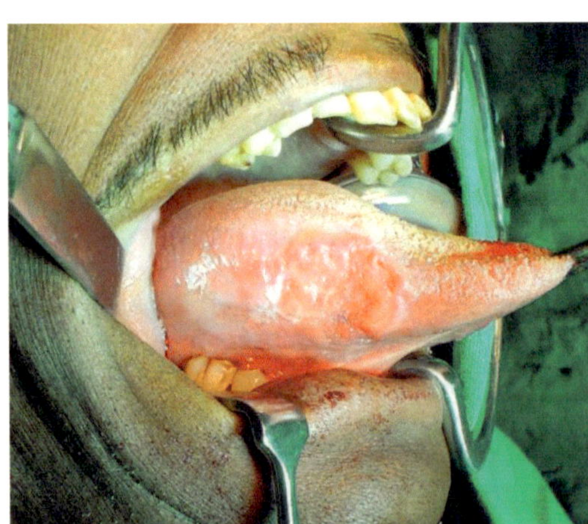

Figure 1. Resection of squamous cell carcinoma of right lateral border of tongue by per oral approach.

Lower cheek flap: This approach allows access to the mandible, lower gingiva-buccal complex, retro-molar trigone and tonsil. Depending upon the location and extent of the tumor, the decision to preserve the metal nerve and the lateral mandibular periosteum is made.

Mandibulotomy: This approach allows access to the posterior tongue, tonsil and soft palate. A paramedian mandibulotomy is preferred between the lateral incisor and canine since these teeth roots are maximally divergent. Care should be taken to remain anterior to the mental nerve. A step ladder osteotomy offers a better mechanical advantage.

Pull through: This approach is often employed for large volume tongue cancers with extension into the hyoglossus muscle provided gingivolingual mucosa and alveolus are free.

Commando approach: This terminology has fallen out of favor and the term composite resections are used to denote excision of tongue, tonsil and mandible.

2.1.1.2. Subsite specific salient features

Tongue/floor of mouth:

- Aggressive biological behavior
- Notorious for neural and lymphovascular invasion
- Tendency for submucosal spread
- Propensity for nodal and distant metastases
- Depth of invasion and extrinsic tongue muscle involvement bad prognosticators
- Compartmental excisions are recommended for deep invasion of extrinsic tongue musculature to ensure removal of the tumor along with the in-transit lymphatics and contiguous lymph nodal station [7].
- Since reconstruction has direct impact on speech and swallow, following principles must be borne in mind
    - Preserve tip
    - Maintain bulk posteriorly to prevent aspiration
    - Palatal contact to promote better consonant pronunciation
    - Prevent tethering to mandible/inter-dental stitches that will hamper with mobility

Buccal mucosa/gingivobuccal sulcus/mandible:

- High prevalence in Indian subcontinent due to habit of chewed tobacco consumption
- Extent of disease into the masticator space and infra-temporal fossa must be assessed on pre-operative imaging
- Caution should be exercised in estimating deeper soft tissue extent in the setting of trismus and posteriorly located tumors particularly with involvement of the retro-molar trigone area.
- Proximity to and involvement of mandible determines bony resection

- Reconstruction of middle third should be necessarily with free osteocutaneous flaps
- Reconstruction of posterior segment can be with osteocutaneous or soft tissue flaps depending upon age of the patient, disease extent and amount of remnant mandibular segment.
- Placement of the incision (midline or commissure split incision) should be based on anterior extent of the resection margin.

2.1.1.3. Management of mandible

Indications for marginal mandibulectomy:

1. For achieving adequate margin (tumor close to but not involving mandible)
2. Superficial bony erosion
3. Superficial periosteal invasion

However, a mandibular height of minimum 1 cm is essential for bony support after marginal mandibulectomy. In situations where inferior soft tissue or bony margin does not allow this, a segmental mandibulectomy should be contemplated. Soft tissue margins are often used as surrogates to decide bony margins. Frozen section analysis of the bone marrow can alternatively be used to decide adequacy of the same [8].

Indications for segmental mandibulectomy:

1. Gross bony erosion
2. Prior radiation
3. Edentulous mandible
4. Gross paramandibular disease

2.1.1.3.1. Lip

- Squamous cancers are the most common histology
- Involvement of oral commissure has direct bearing on its esthetic and functional performance
- While reconstruction it is important to remember that the lip should have sensation, motion, prevent drooling, permit speech and have a reasonable cosmetic appearance (**Figure 2**).

2.1.1.3.2. Hard palate

- Salivary gland malignancies are common although squamous cancers still remain the most common histology
- Nasal endoscopy should be performed to determine extension into the nasopharyngeal surface of the soft palate.

- For maxillary cancers extending onto hard palate, a hypothetical line extending from the medial canthus to the angle of mandible differentiates inferomedial and superolateral tumors. The former is said to have a significantly better prognosis than the later.

2.1.2. *Management of neck nodes*

An elective neck dissection is now standard of care for all oral cancers [9]. The risk of regional metastases has been correlated to thickness of the tumor, site, size and histological features of the primary [10]. The dissemination of metastatic cancer to regional lymph nodes from primary cancers in the oral cavity occurs in a predictable and sequential fashion [11]. The initial spread from oral cancer occurs at Levels I, II, III. Involvement of Level IV is often implicated in tongue cancers. Isolated skip metastases to Level V are exceedingly uncommon. Some authors propose level IIa positivity as a guide to proceed for level IIB/V clearance [12]. A selective (supraomohyoid) neck dissection clearing Levels I, II, III, and IV is considered appropriate for most primary oral cancers with clinico-radiologically N0 neck [13]. The extent and of neck dissection varies according to the clinico-radiological staging of nodal disease (**Table 3**). Sentinel node biopsy has gained much interest as a reliable and oncologically safe, less morbid alternative to elective neck dissection [14]. However, requirement of resources and expertise and a reasonably steep learning curve for accurate interpretation of results has limited its wider applicability.

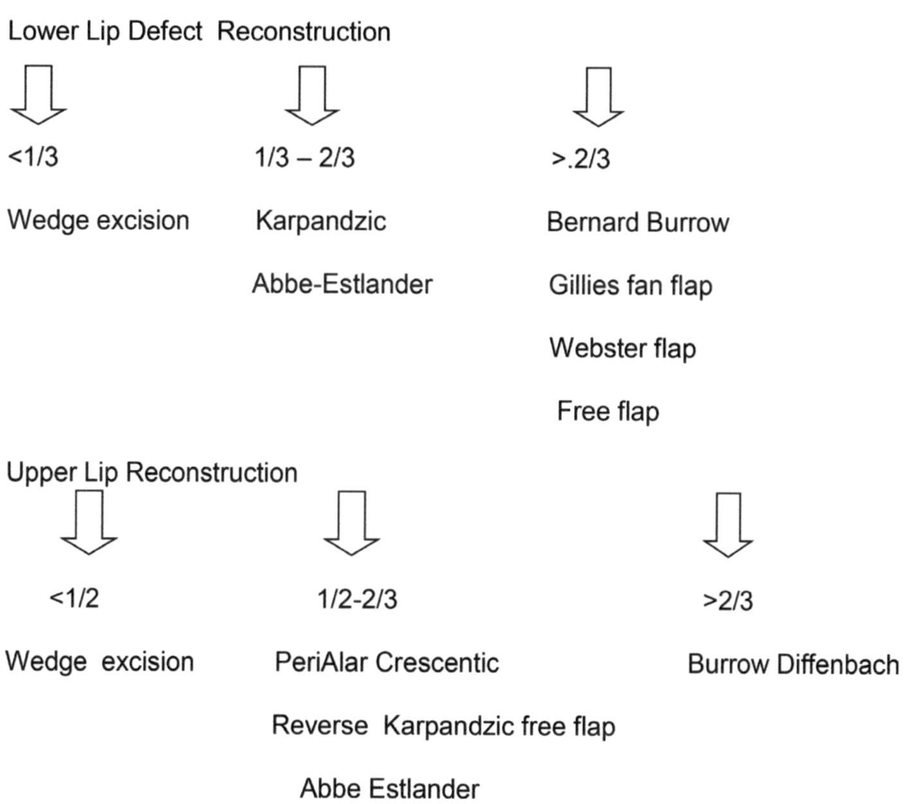

Figure 2. Techniques for reconstruction of upper and lower lip defects.

2.1.2.1. Incisions for neck dissection

The exact location and type of skin incision will depend on the site of the primary tumor and whether a unilateral or bilateral neck dissection is planned. Caution should be exercised to avoid tri-pointer suturing over the great vessels to safeguard from a dreaded complication of carotid blow-out. Triangular edges in the flaps are liable to undergo ischemic necrosis and should be similarly avoided. The vertical limbs in the incision should be avoided as they produce unsightly scars and contractures which produce neck morbidity.

The following are the various routinely employed incisions used for neck dissection [15, 16].

I. Macfee incision

II. Crile's incision

III. Hay-Martin's incision

IV. Schobinger's incision

V. Modified Conley's incision

VI. Apron incision

VII. Modified Macfee incision

2.1.3. Reconstruction

Reconstruction after oral cancer surgery should aim at restoration of both form and function. The principle of "like for like" is a good rationale for deciding the type of reconstruction. This can be accomplished by the following: (1) primary closure, (2) split thickness skin graft, (3) vascularized cutaneous free flap, (4) regional myocutaneous flap, or (5) microvascular free

N_0	1. Selective neck dissection (**Figure 3**) 2. Frozen section/crush imprint cytology for clinically suspicious nodes-SOS modified neck dissection
N+	Modified neck dissection (**Figure 4**)
Classical radical neck dissection [13, 14]	1. N3 disease 2. Gross invasion of the spinal accessory nerve/internal jugular vein/sternocleidomastoid 3. Recurrent or persistent metastatic carcinoma after previous radiation therapy, chemoradiation therapy, or previous selective neck dissection
Extended radical neck dissection	1. Gross extranodal disease. 2. Involvement of the skin or platysma. 3. Involvement of other nonlymphatic structures like great vessels (carotid), nerves (vagus, phrenic, sympathetic plexus, etc.) muscles of neck, mandible, maxilla, infratemporal fossa, sinuses, etc.

Table 3. Extent of neck dissection for oral cancers.

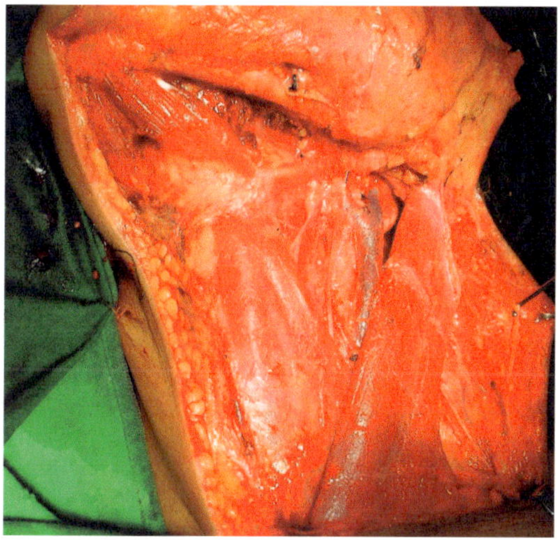

Figure 3. Selective neck dissection preserving greater auricular nerve, sternocleidomastoid muscle (SCM), internal jugular vein (IJV), spinal accessory nerve (SAN).

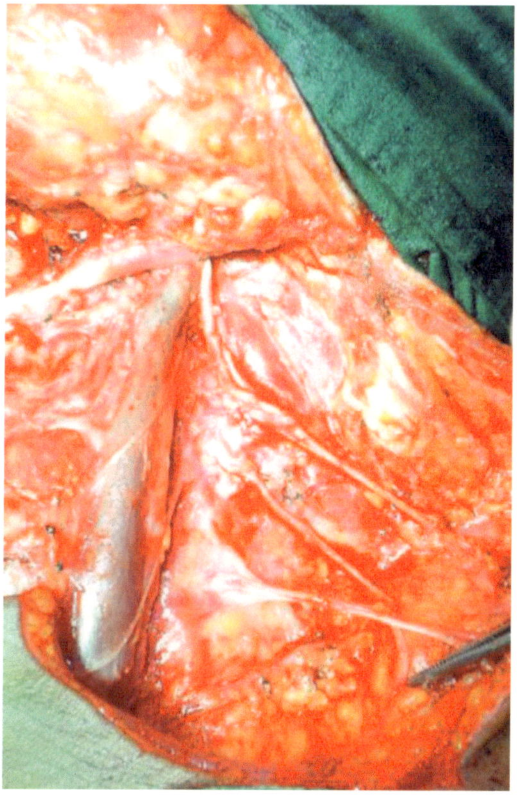

Figure 4. Modified radical neck dissection preserving IJV, SAN and sacrificing SCM.

flap. A variety of free flaps consisting of skin, muscle, bone, or any combination of these tissues are available for reconstruction in the oral cavity. There is an increasing inclination towards microvascular reconstructions for oral resections in light of better functional and cosmetic outcomes [17]. To summarize, the choice of reconstruction should be guided by the anticipated postoperative morbidity, extent of resection and the available infrastructure, resources and expertise.

2.1.3.1. Tongue

Being a very mobile organ and of paramount importance in deglutition and prevention of aspiration, reconstruction of tongue defects is a challenge (**Table 4**).

2.1.3.2. Gingivobuccal-alveolus complex

Smaller defects can be closed with local flaps such as palatal, buccal fat pad, posterior tongue flap, nasolabial flap, etc. Larger soft tissue defects should be reconstructed with FRAFF, FALT or PMMC and deltopectoral flaps depending on defect, disease and patient factors and the expertise available. Segmental mandibular defects should ideally be reconstructed with free osteocutaneous flaps like the fibular, iliac crest, scapular flap, etc. Posterior mandibular defects in old age patients can be considered for PMMC flap reconstruction. Hard palate defects can be reconstructed with dental obturators or osteocutaneous flaps.

2.2. Radiotherapy

Radiotherapy has undergone remarkable advances in the past few decades. With the advent of intensity modulated radiotherapy and image guided radiotherapy, radiation treatment delivery has become very precise with minimum damage of surrounding areas at risk [18]. Tumors of the tongue require bilateral face and neck radiation whereas buccal complex tumors warrant unilateral face and neck radiation. The primary role of radiotherapy in oral cancers is in the adjuvant setting. Upfront radiation is offered in very select cases of early small size accessible tumors (generally brachytherapy) or as a non-surgical treatment for locally advanced cancers where either surgery is contra-indicated on medical grounds.

<30% substance loss	Primary closure (some surgeons also consider leaving behind a raw surface for very superficial small size defects)
>30% tissue loss	1. Free radial artery forearm flap (FRAFF) Supple, sensate 2. Pectoralis major myocutaneous flap (PMMC)/ Free anterolateral thigh flap (FALT)/ Rectus abdominis flap Provide good bulk

Table 4. Reconstruction of tongue defects.

Indications for adjuvant radiation:

- T_3/T_4 disease
- Positive nodal metastases/multiple positive lymph nodes (>2 lymph nodes)/bilateral positive lymph nodes
- Extranodal invasion
- Poor differentiation
- Adverse pathological factors such as lymphovascular or perineural invasion
- Positive surgical margins
- Recurrent tumors

Indications for adjuvant chemoradiation [19]:

- Positive surgical margins
- Perinodal extension

Some oncologists practice concurrent chemoradiation for bulky or level IV/V nodal disease or T_3/T_4 tumors, lymphovascular or perineural invasion also [20, 21].

2.2.1. Brachytherapy

Interstitial brachytherapy represents a traditional approach for OSCC and is an alternative to external beam radiotherapy (EBRT). Brachytherapy delivers radiotherapy by positioning radioactive sources in direct proximity to the tumor target area. Brachytherapy is a feasible treatment option restricted to following conditions in oral malignancies:

- Superficial lesions (especially over lip, tip of nose where surgical resection will lead to considerable cosmetic deformity)
- Small tumors
- Tumors away from bone
- N0 nodal status

2.3. Chemotherapy

Chemotherapy has no curative potential in oral cancers.

2.3.1. Neo-adjuvant chemotherapy (NACT)

For selected T4 tumors where morbidity of resection is extremely high, NACT can be administered. Induction chemotherapy has been used as a biological decider for locally advanced borderline operable disease [22].

However, in candidates that undergo surgery, it must be borne in mind that resection margins must be planned taking into account the initial extent of the tumor and not the measurements of the shrunken tumor after NACT.

2.3.2. Palliative chemotherapy

Combination palliative chemotherapy has been documented to prolong progression free survival by few months. However, the risk benefit ratio of the disease response and systemic side effects of the chemotherapy must be critically evaluated at each stage to decide regarding continual treatment.

3. Conclusions

Oral cancer is primarily a surgically managed disease. However, treatment needs to be personalized based on subsite, stage and biology of tumor, patient health profile and the infrastructure and expertise available. Appropriate management of cervical nodal metastases has a direct bearing on prognosis. Reconstructive options must be tailored to suit patient needs in order to regain as much as possible form and function. Adjuvant treatment adherence and regular follow-up in the surveillance period should be adhered to.

4. Future prospects

PDL1 (programmed death ligand) antagonists are gaining promise as an alternative for recurrent and metastatic head and neck cancers [23]. Targeting the m TOR pathway for exploring resistance to Cetuximab is established [24]. Research and interest in Immunotherapy is also increasing however, it is still only in an experimental phase.

Author details

Neeti Kapre Gupta[1,2,3*], Monica Mahajan[1,2,4] and Apeksha Hore[1,5]

*Address all correspondence to: hi.neeti@gmail.com

1 Neeti Clinics, Nagpur, India

2 Tata Memorial Hospital, Mumbai, India

3 International Federation of Head and Neck Oncologic Societies, UK

4 SDKS Dental College, Nagpur, India

5 VSPM Dental College, Nagpur, India

References

[1] Shah J. Head and Neck Surgery and Oncology. 3rd ed. St. Louis, MO: Mosby; 2003

[2] Mohiyuddin SMA, Padiyar BV, Suresh TN, et al. Clinicopathological study of surgical margins in squamous cell carcinoma of buccal mucosa. World Journal of Otorhinolaryngology—Head and Neck Surgery. 2016;**2**(1):17-21

[3] Byers RM, Bland KI, Borlase B, Luna M. The prognostic and therapeutic value of frozen section determinations in the surgical treatment of squamous carcinoma of the head and neck. American Journal of Surgery. 1978;**136**(4):525-528

[4] van den Hoogen FJ, Manni JJ. Value of the supraomohyoid neck dissection with frozen section analysis as a staging procedure in the clinically negative neck in squamous cell carcinoma of the oral cavity. European Archives of Oto-Rhino-Laryngology. 1992;**249**(3):144-148

[5] Chaturvedi P, Datta S, Nair S, Nair D, Pawar P, Vaishampayan S, et al. Gross examination by the surgeon as an alternative to frozen section for assessment of adequacy of surgical margin in head and neck squamous cell carcinoma. Head & Neck. 2014;**36**(4):557-563

[6] http://www.jhnps.org. IP: 49.248.194.11

[7] Calabrese L, Bruschini R, Giugliano G, Ostuni A, Maffini F, Massaro MA, et al. Compartmental tongue surgery: Long term oncologic results in the treatment of tongue cancer. Oral Oncology. 2011;**47**(3):174-179

[8] Namin AW, Bruggers SD, Panuganti BA, Christopher KM, Walker RJ, Varvares MA. Efficacy of bone marrow cytologic evaluations in detecting occult cancellous invasion. The Laryngoscope. 2015;**125**(5):E173-E179

[9] D'Cruz AK, Vaish R, Kapre N, et al. Elective versus therapeutic neck dissection in node-negative oral cancer. The New England Journal of Medicine. 2015;**373**(6):521-529

[10] Spiro RH, Huvos AG, Gy W, et al. Predictive value of tumor thickness in squamous cancer confined to the tongue and floor of mouth. American Journal of Surgery. 1986;**152**:345-350

[11] Shah JP. Patterns of nodal metastasis from squamous cell carcinomas of the upper aerodigestive tract. American Journal of Surgery. 1990;**160**:405-409

[12] Pantvaidya GH, Pal P, Vaidya AD, Pai PS, D'Cruz AK. Prospective study of 583 neck dissections in oral cancers: Implications for clinical practice. Head and Neck. 2014;**36**(10):1503-1507

[13] Brazilian Head and Neck Cancer Study Group. Results of a prospective trial of elective modified radical classical versus supraomohyoid neck dissection in the management of oral squamous cell carcinoma. American Journal of Surgery. 1996;**176**:422-427

[14] Schilling C, Stoeckli SJ, Haerle SK, et al. Sentinel European Node Trial (SENT): 3-year results of sentinel node biopsy in oral cancer. European Journal of Cancer. 2015;**51**(18):2777-2784

[15] Shah J. Surgical approaches to the oral cavity primary and neck. International Journal of Radiation Oncology, Biology, Physics. 2007;**69**(2(Suppl)):S15-S18

[16] Susan D et al. Radical neck dissection. Operative Techniques in Otolaryngology. 2004;**15**:152-159

[17] Urken ML, Buchbinder D, Weinberg H, Vickery C, Sheiner A, Parker R, et al. Functional evaluation following microvascular oromandibular reconstruction of the oral cancer patient: A comparative study of reconstructed and nonreconstructed patients. The Laryngoscope. 2015;**125**(7):1512

[18] Nutting CM, Morden JP, Harrington KJ, et al. Parotid-sparing intensity modulated versus conventional radiotherapy in head and neck cancer (PARSPORT): A phase 3 multicentre randomised controlled trial. The Lancet Oncology. 2011;**12**(2):127-136

[19] Bernier J, Cooper JS. Chemoradiation after surgery for high-risk head and neck cancer patients: How strong is the evidence? The Oncologist. 2005;**10**(3):215-224

[20] Bernier J, Domenge C, Ozsahin M, et al. Postoperative irradiation with or without concomitant chemotherapy for locally advanced head and neck cancer. The New England Journal of Medicine. 2004;**350**(19):1945-1952

[21] Cooper JS, Pajak TF, Forastiere AA, et al. Postoperative concurrent radiotherapy and chemotherapy for high-risk squamous-cell carcinoma of the head and neck. The New England Journal of Medicine. 2004;**350**(19):1937-1944

[22] Patil VM, Prabhash K, Noronha V, et al. Neoadjuvant chemotherapy followed by surgery in very locally advanced technically unresectable oral cavity cancers. Oral Oncology. 2014;**50**(10):1000-1004

[23] Seiwert TY, Burtness B, Mehra R, et al. Safety and clinical activity of pembrolizumab for treatment of recurrent or metastatic squamous cell carcinoma of the head and neck (KEYNOTE-012): An open-label, multicentre, phase 1b trial. The Lancet Oncology. 2016;**17**(7):956-965

[24] Wang Z, Martin D, Molinolo AA, et al. mTOR co-targeting in cetuximab resistance in head and neck cancers harboring PIK3CA and RAS mutations. Journal of the National Cancer Institute. 2014;**106**(9):pii:dju215. DOI: 10.1093/jnci/dju215. Print Sep 2014

Chapter 6

The Mechanisms of Proliferation and Energy Metabolism in Oral Cancer

Masakatsu Fukuda and Hideaki Sakashita

Additional information is available at the end of the chapter

http://dx.doi.org/10.5772/intechopen.87091

Abstract

Human oral squamous cell carcinoma (HOSCC) is the most common head and neck malignant neoplasm. Therapy is generally performed in multidisciplinary approach that used chemotherapy, radiotherapy, and surgery against patients with oral cancer; however, we cannot avoid dysfunction due to its side effects or surgical defects, and it significantly impacts the postoperative quality of life, unfortunately. Therefore, a better understanding of the molecular mechanisms driving oral carcinogenesis may lead to new diagnostic and therapeutic approaches to this disease and improve the prognosis of HOSCC patients. Cancer cells process a fundamental change in its bioenergetics metabolism from normal cells on an altered glucose and lipid metabolism. Recent insights into tumor metabolism have further revealed that oncogenic signaling pathways directly promote metabolic reprogramming to upregulate biosynthesis of lipids, carbohydrates, protein, DNA, and RNA, leading to enhanced growth of tumors. Therefore, targeting cell metabolism has become a novel direction for drug development in oncology. Moreover, molecular mechanisms causing these metabolic changes are just starting to be unraveled. This chapter presents recent findings on molecular markers that have been involved in the mechanisms of proliferation and energy metabolism of oral cancer and in addition provides new perspectives on oral cancer diagnosis and treatments.

Keywords: oral cancer, squamous cell carcinoma (SCC), cell adhesion molecules (CAMs), cytokines, anticancer agents, energy metabolism (glycolysis and lipid)

1. Introduction

Cancer development and fatality are gradually increasing worldwide. It is thought that the reasons are complex but associated with both aging and increase in the population [1, 2].

With the rapid global population increase and aging, the rising significance of cancer as a leading cause of death is partly correlated with a marked decline in mortality rates due to stroke and coronary heart disease in many countries. In addition, tobacco and alcohol consumption are known to be etiologically associated with carcinogenesis. Cancer is both a genetic and progressively systemic disease. In all types of cancer, somatic cells begin to divide uncontrollably and spread into surrounding tissues. Cancer cells can arise almost anywhere in the human body. Normal cells grow and divide according to the body's needs, and when they age or become damaged, they die and are replaced by new cells. However, when cancer arises, this orderly process breaks down: as cellular abnormalities increase, old or damaged cells survive rather than being removed, and new cells form when they are not needed. These extra cells can divide uncontrollably and may form malignant tumors. Although many cancers form solid tumors composed of masses of tissue, cancers of the blood, such as leukemias, generally do not form solid tumors [2–4]. Head and neck cancer is a common neoplasm that encompasses epithelial malignant tumors of the nasopharynx, larynx, and mouth, representing about 6% of all cases and accounting for an estimated over 650,000 new cancer cases and over 350,000 cancer-related deaths worldwide every year [5, 6]. Oral cancer is the most notably frequent cancer type in the head and neck region, squamous cell carcinoma being the most common single entity. Oral cancers comprise two categories: those affecting the oral cavity (lips, inner lips, cheeks, teeth, gums, the anterior two-thirds of the tongue, the floor, and palate) and those affecting the oropharynx (middle region of the throat, including the tonsils and base of the tongue). Such cancers may arise in any location, although there are certain areas that are affected more frequently, such as the tongue and gingiva. These areas represent about 90% of all malignancies of the oral cavity [7, 8]. However, despite significant advances in surgery and chemotherapy over the last few decades [9], oral cancer is still characterized by a poor prognosis and a low survival rate [10]. The 5-year survival rate of those diagnosed is ~ 60%.

In patients diagnosed with oral cancers at an advanced stage, there is a high incidence of metastasis to surrounding tissues, lymph nodes, and distant organs [5]. Metastasis is recognized as a process, whereby genetic instability in the primary tumor accelerates cell heterogeneity, allowing a few metastatic clones to eventually emerge and be positively selected to disseminate cancer at a distance [11]. This is the most annihilating stage of malignancy and the leading cause of cancer-related death. In metastasis, cancer cells break away from the primary cancer, travel through the blood or lymph system, and form new metastatic tumors elsewhere in the body. Each metastatic tumor is the same type of cancer as the primary tumor [12, 13], and the cells of each resemble each other upon microscopic observation. Moreover, they usually share common molecular features, such as the presence of specific genetic changes. It is clear that only a minority of malignant cells participate in the process of metastasis, due to interaction with host tissues and the intrinsic characteristics of the cancer cells themselves; thus, metastasis may imply an escape of these cells from the hostile environment they have created, characterized by features such as hypoxia, inflammation, and immunological surveillance [14–16].

This chapter details recent findings on molecular markers that are involved in the mechanisms of proliferation and energy metabolism of oral cancer and provides new perspectives on its diagnosis and treatments.

2. Role of cell adhesion molecules (CAMs) in proliferation of oral cancer

CAMs are typically single-pass transmembrane receptors [17] compounded of three stored domains: an intracellular domain that interacts with a transmembrane domain, an extracellular domain, and the cytoskeleton. These domains can interact in several different ways [18]. The first way is through homophilic binding, where the same CAMs bind to each other. They are also capable of heterophilic binding, which means a CAM on one cell will bind to different CAMs on another cell. The third type of binding is that between cells and substrate, where a mutual extracellular ligand binds two different CAMs. There are four major superfamilies, or groups, of CAMs: the immunoglobulin super family of cell adhesion molecules (IgCAMs), the cadherins, the integrins, and the c-type lectin-like domain proteins (CTLDs). Proteoglycans are also believed to be a class of CAMs. One classification system involves distinction between calcium-dependent and calcium-independent CAMs [19]. The Ig-superfamily CAMs and integrins are not dependent on calcium ions, whereas selectins and cadherins are calcium-dependent. In addition, integrins participate in cell-matrix interactions, while other CAM families play some important roles in cell-to-cell interactions [20].

2.1. Neural cell adhesion molecule (NCAM)

Neural cell adhesion molecule (NCAM) is a family of cell surface glycoproteins playing an important role in the development of the nervous system, fasciculation, axonal outgrowth, regulation of cell migration, and branching [21]. NCAM has several isoforms derived from alternative splicing of a single gene [22–24]. In particular, the three major isoforms with molecular weights of 120, 140, and 180 kDa have similar extracellular parts but differ in the disposition of their domains, which are cytoplasmic for the two larger polypeptides [25, 26]. Furthermore, the expression of NCAM is upregulated by transforming growth factor (TGF)-β1 [27–29]. Although NCAM was initially considered to exist only in neural tissue, it has since been observed in the human kidney, lung, fetal muscle, and colon, as well as in elements of the hemopoietic system. Furthermore, it has been described that NCAM is expressed by a variety of human tumors and associated with perineural invasion by various neoplasms, such as gallbladder cancer, melanoma, bile duct cancer, and adenoid cystic carcinoma of the head and neck [30–35]. We have also demonstrated previously that NCAM is sporadically found in the adenoid cystic carcinoma, derived from human submandibular salivary gland, *in vivo* [36]. NCAM is believed to mediate adhesion between cells through a calcium ion-independent homophilic (NCAM-NCAM) binding mechanism and to mediate adhesion between neurons and the extracellular matrix through heterophilic binding (NCAM to another ligand or counter-receptor) [21]. It has been described that exogenously added NCAM can inhibit the proliferation of cultured neonatal astrocytes and of astrocytes responding to a penetrating lesion in the adult rat brain, *in vivo* [37, 38], suggesting that these effects are mediated by homophilic binding to NCAM on the astrocyte membrane.

Adenoid cystic carcinoma (ACC) is a well-known and typical malignant salivary gland tumor. ACCs are biologically aggressive and can bring metastases even when many years have passed after excision of the primary tumor. Facial paralysis is especially frequent, causing perineural and/or neural invasion. We have attempted to examine the role of NCAM by investigating the effect of anti-NCAM antibody (MAb NCAM) and TGF-β1 in human salivary gland tumor cells. The expression and distribution of NCAM were also investigated in ACC tissues. We further found that apoptotic cell death was induced via a DNA damage signal through the mitochondria, inducing release of cytochrome *c* into the cytoplasm of salivary gland tumor cells [36]. However, MAb NCAM had no effect on human oral squamous cell carcinoma (HOSCC) cell lines, which do not express NCAM. As shown in **Figure 1**, these results indicate that the effect of MAb NCAM is specific to NCAM-expressing tumor cells, such as human salivary gland tumor cells; furthermore, blocking the ability of NCAM through MAb NCAM, as well as the homophilic (NCAM-NCAM) binding mechanism, rather than regulating a signaling pathway of cell proliferation, may in fact induce a negative signal such as apoptosis in human salivary gland tumor cells. In addition, homophilic (NCAM-NCAM) binding may activate multiple signaling pathways that differ among cell types. In view of the fact that NCAM expression on human salivary gland tumor cells is upregulated by TGF-β1, it can be hypothesized that a further homophilic (NCAM-NCAM) binding mechanism may be activated and that consequently the proliferative activity of HSG cells may also be upregulated by TGF-β1-mediated NCAM activity (**Figure 2**).

On the other hand, cimetidine, the most studied histamine type-2 receptor (H2R) antagonist used clinically, is commonly prescribed to treat gastroesophageal reflux disease as well as

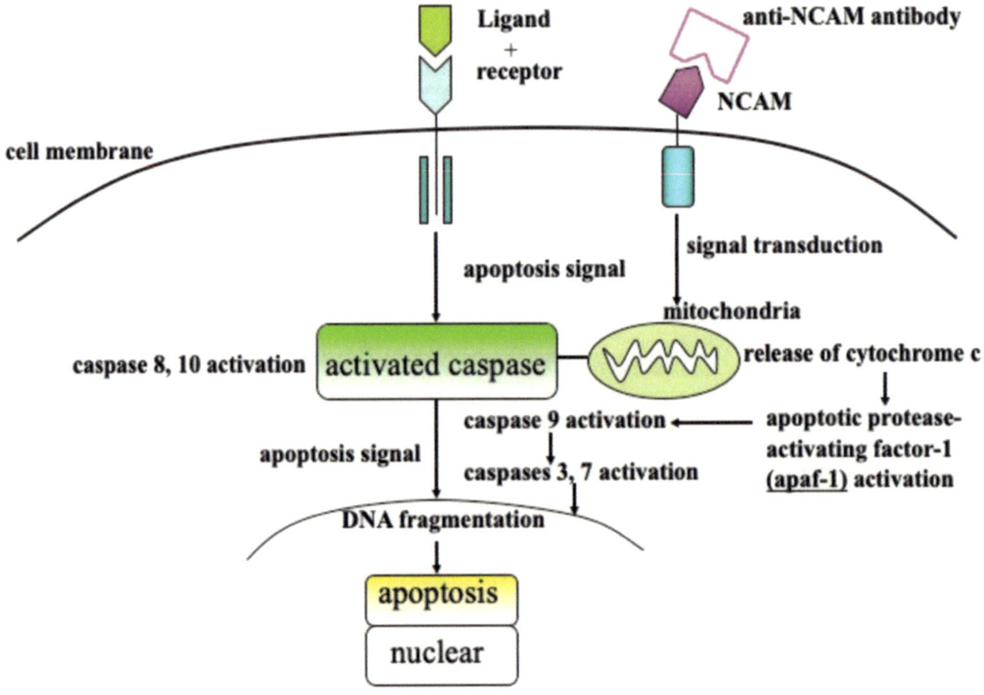

Figure 1. Schematic representation of MAb NCAM-induced apoptotic signal transduction pathways via the DNA damage signal through the mitochondria involved in apaf-1 and caspase activation in NCAM-expressing cells.

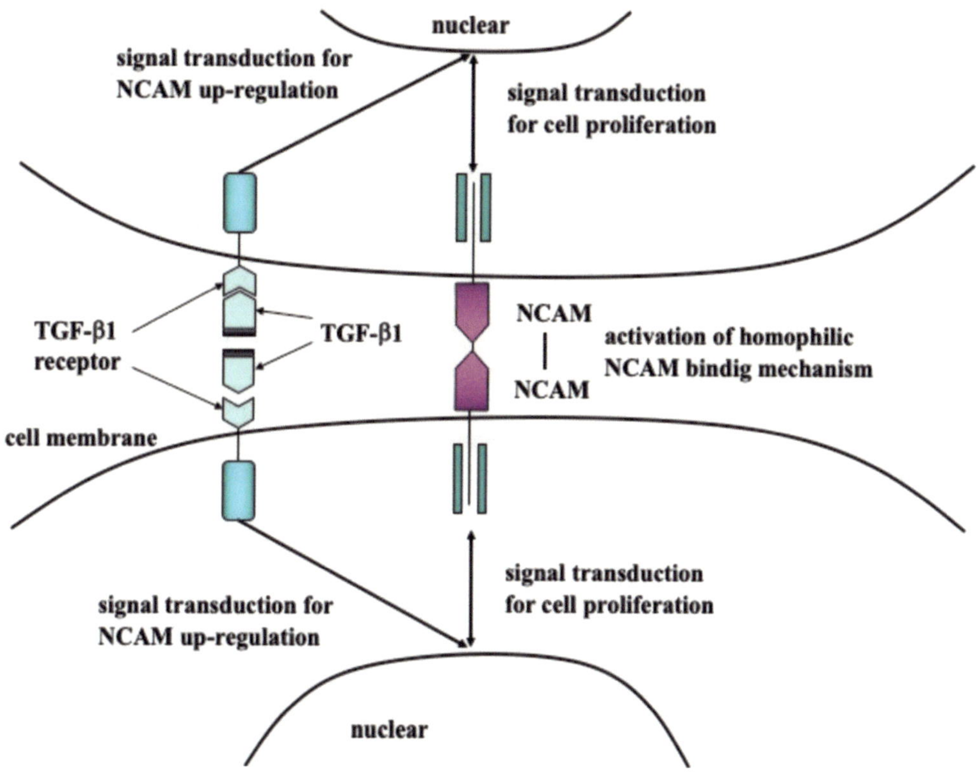

Figure 2. Schematic representation of TGF-β1-induced upregulation of NCAM expression and proliferative activity involved in homophilic (NCAM-NCAM) binding mechanism in NCAM-expressing cells.

gastric and duodenal ulcers [39]. Cimetidine has recently been shown to possess antitumor activity against gastric, kidney, and colon cancers, as well as melanomas [40–43]. A recent study has suggested that this behavior of cimetidine is mediated through three different effects: a direct inhibitory effect on tumor growth by blocking the cell growth activity of histamine via activation of H2 receptors and an indirect effect involving inhibition of tumor-associated angiogenesis, an immunomodulatory effect through augmentation of the host's immune response to tumor cells, and an inhibitory effect on cancer cell migration and adhesion to endothelial cells, thus inhibiting tumor angiogenesis and metastasis [44]. We have also examined the NCAM-associated impact of cimetidine on tumor growth and perineural/neural invasion in salivary gland tumors using an in vitro cell culture system and an *in vivo* nude mouse cancer model. These experiments clearly indicated that cimetidine effectively downregulated the expression of NCAM by inhibiting NF-κB transactivation, subsequently blocking salivary gland tumor cell adhesion to neural cells, and ultimately inducing apoptosis in salivary gland tumor cells, thus preventing the growth of salivary gland tumor masses in nude mice [45]. Although malignant glandular tumors are commonly known to be resistant to chemotherapy and/or radiation, the clinical application of cimetidine as an anticancer drug might provide an integral part of future therapeutic strategies against NCAM-expressing tumors such as adenoid cystic carcinoma.

Finally, it was suggested that NCAM might be associated with not only a cell-to-cell adhesion mechanism but also tumorigenesis, including the occurrence, development, and perineural/neural invasion of human salivary gland tumors.

Further studies will be required to identify the signal transduction pathways by which treatment with cimetidine suppresses the growth of salivary gland tumors and to establish a strategy for cimetidine-based therapy for those tumors.

2.2. Coxsackievirus and adenovirus receptor (CAR/CXADR)

Coxsackievirus and adenovirus receptor (CAR/CXADR), a transmembrane glycoprotein, was initially characterized as a viral attachment site on the surface of epithelial cells (**Figure 3**) [46]. Later it was identified as a component of the tight junction (TJ) complex, an interacting partner for a number of other TJ proteins and a regulator of TJ formation [47–52]. Furthermore, CAR is known to be a cell-cell adhesion molecule [53, 54]. In terms of function, loss of CAR has been considered to diminish intercellular adhesion, increase proliferation, and promote the migration as well as invasion of cancer cells [55, 56]. On the basis of these observations, a tumor-suppressive role of CAR in human cancers has speculated. Although it has recently been described [55–58] that CAR is observed in various organs, it is still unclear whether it is expressed in oral cancer. Therefore, we examined the role of CAR in SCC in the oral cavity (data not shown). This revealed that CAR was constitutively expressed in five oral SCC cell lines. To analyze the function of CAR, we then examined the proliferative activity of SAS cells

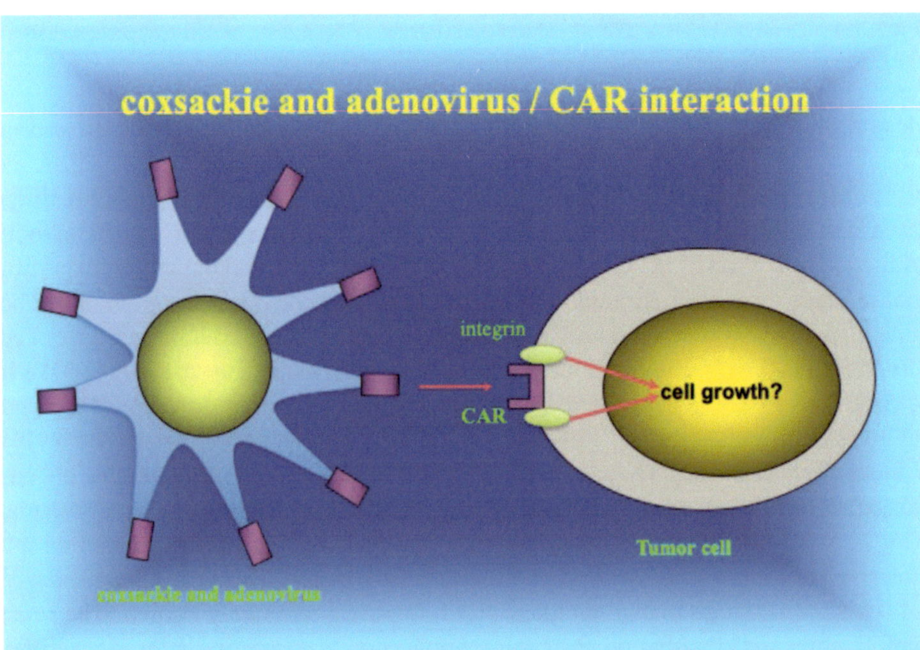

Figure 3. Schematic representation of coxsackievirus and adenovirus receptor on the tumor cells.

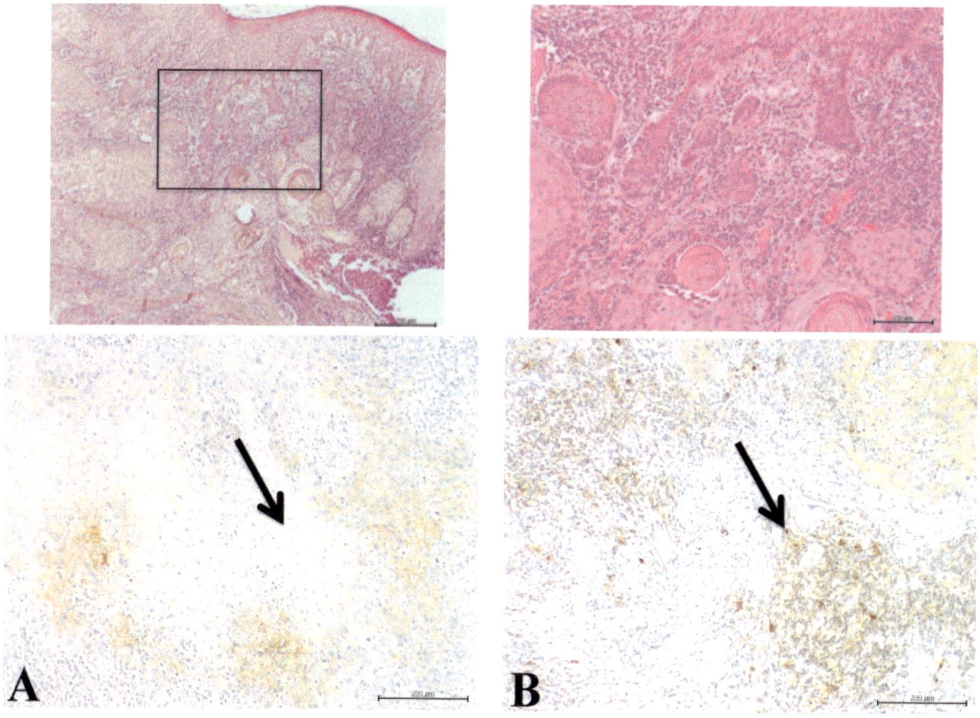

Figure 4. (A) The positive reaction for PAb CAR was observed on the membrane of tumor cells in 19 of 40 cases (47.5%) of SCCs. (B) NF-κB immunoreactivity were clearly detected in 30 of 40 cases (100%) in the HOSCC tissues. The immunoreactivity for CAR especially tended to fade away in the invasive front of oral SCC tissues. NF-kappaB (+)/CAR (−), 15/21 cases (71.4%).

after *CAR* gene knockdown. However, *CAR* knockdown did not promote the proliferative activity of SAS cells. Although the expression level of CAR was decreased by *CAR* knockdown, that of NF-κB p65 (RelA) showed little change. Furthermore, SAS cell numbers were notably reduced by CAR overexpression. Finally, it was suggested that the overexpression of CAR in SAS cells led to apoptosis via activation of caspase-9. In addition, the localizations of CAR and RelA in 40 samples of HOSCC at various stages were investigated using immunohistochemistry. A positive reaction for polyclonal antibody (PAb) CAR was weakly observed on the membrane of carcinoma cells in 19 of 40 cases (47.5%) of HOSCC. The immunoreactivity for CAR further tended to fade at the invasive front of oral SCC (**Figure 4**). In the meantime, RelA immunoreactivity was strongly positive, particularly on the nucleus of carcinoma cells at the invasive front, in 30 of 40 cases (75%) of HOSCC. These observations suggest that CAR plays a significant role in the inhibition of oral cancer cell growth.

3. Role of cytokines in oral cancer cell proliferation

Cytokines are composed of a large family of secreted proteins that bind to and signal through defined cell surface receptors on a wide variety of target cells, playing an important role in the maintenance of homeostasis. Furthermore, many cytokines share structural features and effects during inflammation, development, or immune responses.

The concept of a control mechanism for cellular growth via regulation of apoptosis has recently been erected in a wide variety of tissue systems. Changes in the balance between cell survival and death are definite signs of emergence of various tumors. Therefore, modulation of apoptosis is required so as to maintain the homeostasis of a living organism. The expression of cytokines and their receptors in human oral cancers has attracted a great deal of interest because of their potential importance in tumor immunity. In particular, it has been described that members of the tumor necrosis factor (TNF) family, including Fas/FasL and TNF-related apoptosis-inducing ligand (TRAIL), regulate the deletion of unnecessary immune cells through induction of apoptosis [59–61]. However, despite their expression of these obvious antigens, tumor evasion by the immune system is often inefficient. It is considered that tumor cells may also evade immune attack by expressing TRAIL, Fas ligand, or other molecules that induce apoptosis in activated T cells [62].

3.1. Tumor necrosis factor-related apoptosis-inducing ligand (TRAIL)

TRAIL, also called APO2 ligand (APO2L), is a novel member of the TNF cytokine family that was originally characterized by its ability to induce apoptosis [59, 60]. It is recognized that at least four closely related receptors bind to TRAIL: death receptor-4 (DR4) and DR5/KILLER, which contain cytoplasmic death domains and signal apoptosis [60, 61]; decoy receptor-1 (DcR1) [61–63], which lacks a cytoplasmic tail and inhibits TRAIL function; and DcR2 [64, 65], which contains a cytoplasmic region with a truncated death domain that does not transduce the death signal [67]. TRAIL interacts with its agonistic receptors DR4 and DR5, inducing apoptosis in a wide variety of cancer cell lines derived from breast carcinoma, lung carcinoma, colon carcinoma, lymphoma, malignant melanoma, and malignant glioma [59, 60, 68, 69]. Although DR4 is expressed in many normal human tissues and cells, including spleen and peripheral blood leukocytes, TRAIL induces apoptosis in various cancer cells, but not in normal cells [70]. This may be explained by the fact that TRAIL also interacts with the antagonistic decoy receptors DcR1 and DcR2, which are expressed in normal tissues but not in cancer cells (**Figure 5**) [66, 67]. Neither DcR1 nor DcR2 receptors induce apoptosis, but they protect cells from TRAIL-induced apoptosis [64–66]. Until now, the biological involvement of the complex TRAIL receptor system has remained unclear, and the existing data are conflicting. Nevertheless, because of its selective cytotoxicity against tumor cells, TRAIL is regarded as a promising anticancer weapon that might be highly effective *in vivo* with few side effects, as it has little or no function on normal tissues.

TRAIL is expressed in most normal human cells and tissues, including the peripheral blood leukocytes, spleen, lung, and prostate, but not the brain [60]. However, the expression of TRAIL in human neoplasms is largely unknown. Accordingly, we have examined whether TRAIL and its receptors are expressed in HOSCC tissues or cell lines and whether these cell lines are sensitive to TRAIL-induced apoptosis [71]. This revealed that the mRNA and protein levels of TRAIL and its receptors are co-expressed in HOSCC cell lines in the absence of paracrine fratricide or autocrine suicide. Moreover, TRAIL protein was also detected in 24 of 50

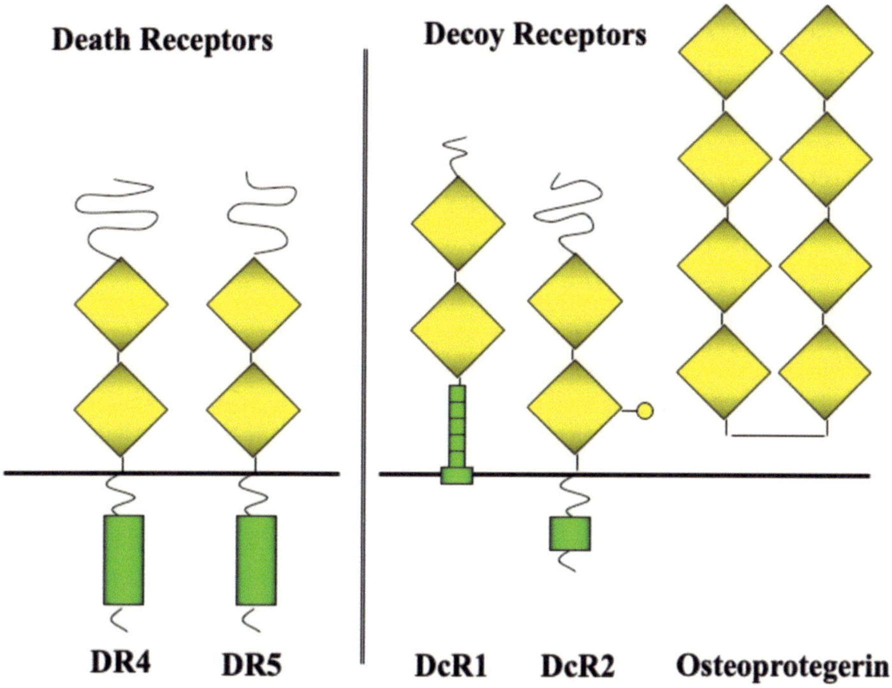

Figure 5. Schematic representation of the death receptors and decoy receptors on the tumor cell.

samples (48%) of HOSCC tissue, and there was no correlation among the WHO grades. These findings suggest that HOSCC has the potential to escape immune surveillance by killing host T lymphocytes via DR4/TRAIL and DR5/TRAIL interactions, as suggested for FasL [72–74].

The expression of decoy receptors in cancer cells is, however, a phenomenon that objects against previous reports [62, 63]. Indeed, several authors have currently described that a decoy receptor is expressed in various cancer types and our results are consistent with their findings [75–77]. Therefore, cancer cells may also avoid TRAIL-induced apoptosis by expressing a decoy receptor.

On the other hand, cells differ significantly in their response to TRAIL. As contrasted to HUVEC or other oral cancer cells, only KB cells undergo significant apoptosis following exposure to recombinant human (rh)TRAIL. The reason why KB cells, despite their expression of a decoy receptor, react to rhTRAIL remains unresolved.

Commonly, the most proximal step in suppression of a death receptor pathway is inhibition of ligand binding. This may be acquired by lack, or the presence of decoy receptors [65–68], or mutations of death receptors [78, 79]. However, it has recently been described that there is no correlation between the expression of TRAIL receptor and susceptibility to TRAIL-induced apoptosis in various cancer types [75–77]. Furthermore, the existence of antiapoptotic proteins, such as bcl-2, bcl-xL, and/or fas-like IL-1-converting enzyme (FLICE)-like inhibitory protein [80, 81], also seems to be significant, as they are resistant to death receptor-mediated apoptosis. Holistically, our results also suggest that there may be no correlation between the expression of TRAIL receptor and sensitivity to TRAIL-induced apoptosis in HOSCC cell lines and that TRAIL-resistant cells (HSC-2, HSC-3, HSC-4, and Ca9-22) may express cytoprotective proteins that block TRAIL-induced apoptosis or that the apoptotic effect of TRAIL is regulated by other mechanisms. It has also been described that TRAIL, in combination with an anticancer drug, acts cooperatively to induce apoptosis in various cancer cells that are resistant to TRAIL or chemotherapy [75, 82, 83]. This combination of TRAIL with chemotherapeutic reagents might be a useful therapeutic strategy against TRAIL-resistant cell lines such as HSC-2, HSC-3, HSC-4, and Ca9-22 used in our investigation.

In fact, we are currently investigating the synergistic effects of α-mangostin and TRAIL on induction of apoptosis via the mitochondrial pathway in squamous cell carcinoma of the oral cavity [84]. To summarize, mangosteen (*Garcinia mangostana*) is a tree discovered in Southeast Asia, and the pericarp of its fruit has been used in folk medicine for the treatment of many human diseases. The rinds of mangosteen fruit contain a high concentration of xanthone, a type of polyphenol. One form of xanthone, α-mangostin, has been described to exhibit chemopreventive effects against chemically induced colon cancer through a decrease of c-Myc expression, suppressing tumor growth in a mouse model of mammary cancer. A recent study has proved the inhibitory effect of α-mangostin on the growth of prostate cancer. However, it is still unclear whether α-mangostin induces cell death in oral cancer. Then, the present study examined the impact of α-mangostin on HOSCC. First, we analyzed the expression of c-Myc in five HOSCC cell lines (HSC-2, HSC-3, HSC-4, Ca9-22, and SAS). The highest level of c-Myc mRNA expression was found in SAS cells and the lowest in HSC-4 cells. Therefore, SAS cells were treated with α-mangostin, which was observed to exert a weak cytocidal effect. Since α-mangostin has been described to exert synergistic effects on cancers when combined with anticancer drugs, we tried to evaluate these synergistic effects of α-mangostin in combination with TRAIL. We found that this combination induced apoptosis in SAS cells through the mitochondrial pathway via activation of caspase-3/caspase-7 and caspase-9, following the release of cytochrome c. In addition, this apoptosis was induced by S/G2/M-phase arrest. Immunoreactivity for c-Myc was revealed in the cytoplasm of cancer cells in 16 (40%) of the 40 cases of HOSCC. These data showed that the combination of α-mangostin and TRAIL may have considerable potential for the treatment of oral cancer.

Further investigation of TRAIL-mediated cell death, including the interaction of TRAIL and its receptors in oral cancer cells under various conditions, will be required to establish a strategy for TRAIL-based oral cancer therapy, which does not cause liver toxicity.

3.2. Hepatocyte growth factor (HGF) and its receptor, c-Met

The tyrosine kinase receptor c-Met ordinarily binds with hepatocyte growth factor (HGF), which triggers its involvement in processes such as cell differentiation, cell growth, angiogenesis, and embryogenesis [85, 86]. However, c-Met activation is also associated with processes related to malignant transformation, such as invasion, tumor growth, angiogenesis, and metastasis [87–91]. In addition to autocrine or paracrine signaling via HGF, c-Met may also be activated via the mutation, protein overexpression or amplification, or transcriptional alteration (via microRNA-mediated dysregulation) of MET [92–94]. c-Met overexpression and MET amplification are thought to be associated with a poorer prognosis in some types of tumors, including non-small cell lung cancer and gastric cancer [94]. In HOSCC, it has also been reported that c-Met expression is associated with cisplatin resistance and a strong propensity for metastasis *in vivo* [95], as well as a poor prognosis [96]. However, details of the involvement of c-Met in oral carcinogenesis are still unclear. Accordingly, we investigated how the relationship between the expression of c-Met and several tumor activation-related markers such as NF-κB is associated with oral carcinogenesis (data not shown). In addition, the expression and distribution of c-Met and NF-κB were also examined in HOSCC tissues (data not shown). The results of real-time qRT-PCR and immunoblot analysis indicated overexpression of c-Met mRNA and protein in SAS cells. Therefore, SAS cells were used in this study. To investigate how c-Met functions in SAS cells, c-Met knockdown analysis was performed. c-Met knockdown appeared to reduce the number of SAS cells. To confirm whether this had been due to apoptosis, caspase activity was then analyzed, and this revealed that apoptosis had indeed occurred via activation of caspases-9 and caspases-3/caspases-7 in SAS by c-Met knockdown. Furthermore, SAS showed cell cycle arrest at S/G2/M phase during this apoptotic cell death. Subsequently, to determine NF-κB expression after c-Met knockdown, we also used a siRNA approach to reduce the expression of c-Met and determine the effects on NF-κB activity. As expected, the level of c-Met mRNA was markedly reduced by c-Met siRNA. Moreover, c-Met knockdown by c-Met siRNA clearly decreased the activation of NF-κB mRNA in SAS cells, in comparison with controls. These data indicated that c-Met upregulated NF-κB activation and consequently that c-Met knockdown led to apoptosis of SAS cells. These combined data suggested that c-Met produced by autologous cancer cells promoted tumor growth. Furthermore, our *in vivo* studies demonstrated c-Met-specific immunoreactivity, consistent with the observation of NF-κB-positive cells in HOSCC biopsy samples (c-Met expression, 9/20 (45%); NF-κB expression, 18/20 cases (90%)). This result suggests that c-Met expression correlates with increased activation of NF-κB. Based on these in vitro and *in vivo* observations, it can be hypothesized that c-Met function leads to NF-κB activation and subsequently anti-apoptosis and that as a consequence, it may be associated with tumorigenesis, including growth, development, and angiogenesis in HOSCC.

Further investigations of the role of c-Met will be required to fully understand c-Met-mediated tumor proliferation and to establish a therapeutic strategy for c-Met-based oral cancer.

4. Energy metabolism in oral cancer

4.1. Glucose metabolism in oral cancer

In normal tissues, adenosine triphosphate (ATP) is mainly produced in mitochondria via complete oxidative phosphorylation (OXPHOS) of glucose. Conversely, only 10% of ATP is produced from glycolysis in which glucose is replaced to lactate [97]. Interestingly, cancer tissues possess high levels of glycolysis in the cytosol even under aerobic conditions, which is upregulated by PI3K/Akt signaling in the mitochondria, a phenomenon known as the "Warburg effect" or "aerobic glycolysis" [98–103]. More than 80 years ago, Otto Warburg

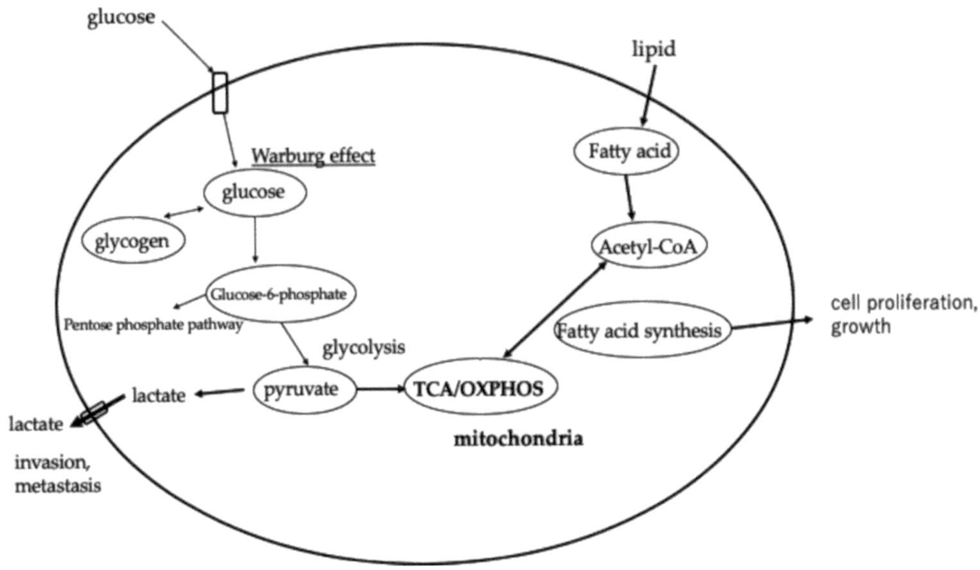

Figure 6. Schematic representation of the connecting glucose and lipid metabolism in cancer cells.

found that cancer cells expended much more glucose to generate lactic acid than normal cells even under conditions of O_2 sufficiency. This finding was the first indication that cancer cells have an alteration of glucose metabolism. Warburg [99] considered that these defects of respiration caused a form of metabolic disturbance that was significant for carcinogenesis. After Warburg, many biologists attempted to clarify the molecular basis of aerobic glycolysis occurring in tumor cells. Accumulated evidence suggested that many cancer-related genes, such as p53, c-Myc, and Ras, are all associated with modulation of the Warburg effect [104]. As a master regulator of the cancer hypoxic response, hypoxia-inducible factor (HIF)-1 plays very important roles in modulating aerobic glycolysis to meet the biosynthetic demands of cancer cells and to protect them from damage due to hypoxic stress [105]. Warburg theorized that cancer cells shift from oxygen-dependent efficient ATP production via OXPHOS in mitochondria to the less efficient cytoplasmic glycolysis. As a result, cancer cells need to burn up more glucose to maintain their energy requirements for survival and growth. It has been reported that HIF-1α activates the expression of glucose transporter 1, 3 (Glut1, Glut3) under hypoxic conditions [106, 107], which acquires sufficient glucose uptake by tumor cells. We also examined HIF, and details can be found in Chapter 10 of the InTech book *Tumor Microenvironment and Myelomonocytic Cells* [108]. Although clarification of glucose metabolism is considered vital for understanding energy metabolism in oral cancer, lipid metabolism has also been receiving attention recently (**Figure 6**).

4.2. Lipid metabolism in oral cancer

Lipids are composed of phospholipids, triglycerides, cholesterol esters, cholesterol, fatty acids, sphingolipids, and other molecules, which are critical components of cellular membranes

[109–113]. In addition to their role as structural components, lipids also act as energy resources and as signaling molecules to sustain cell growth [114–116]. Lipid metabolism is known to be largely altered in cancers [117–120], and worsening lipogenesis has been indicated to be a predominant characteristic of most tumors [114, 115, 121]. In oral cancer, cancer tissues include higher levels of unsaturated fatty acids than those in normal tissue (data not shown). Recent studies have revealed intrinsic molecular alterations in lipid metabolism. Especially, fatty acid synthase (FAS) is a key enzyme for synthesis of fatty acid from acetyl CoA, which is expressed at high levels in the adipose tissue and liver but at low levels in other tissues in humans [122]. FAS is overexpressed in several human cancers, including those of the ovary, bladder, stomach, breast, lung, prostate, oral cavity, and melanoma, and this overexpression is associated with poor prognosis [123, 124]. Furthermore, glutathione peroxidase 4 (GPX4) expression in tumors is positively correlated with tumor survival and linked to pathways that regulate cell proliferation, motility, and tissue remodeling [125]. Knockdown of GPX4 suppresses the formation and progression of cancer and leads to non-apoptotic cell death, ferroptosis. We have also examined the role of GPX4 in HOSCC (data not shown). Ferroptosis is a non-apoptotic form of cell death that can be triggered by conditions or small molecules that inhibit the glutathione-dependent antioxidant enzyme GPX4 or glutathione biosynthesis. This lethal process is defined by depletion of plasma membrane polyunsaturated fatty acids and the iron-dependent accumulation of lipid reactive oxygen species. It has also been reported that GPX4 is negatively regulated by the p53 gene [126]. These data suggest that GPX4 plays a significant role in proliferation and progression and may serve as a potential therapeutic target in HOSCC. Thus, GPX4 would be useful as a predictor of poor outcome in patients with oral cancer, and its antibody might be applicable as an inhibitor of oral cancer progression. Identification of the signaling pathways underlying these events might help to elucidate the mechanism of development of oral cancer. Further investigations into the role of GPX4 will be required to fully understand GPX4-mediated cancer proliferation and to establish a GPX4-based therapeutic strategy for oral cancer.

5. Conclusions

Unlike surgery, chemotherapy, and radiotherapy, which can have serious side effects on the human body, the use of agents that have no such side effects, such as TRAIL, cimetidine, mangostin, and antibodies, for cancer therapy mobilizes and regulates systemic functions, enhancing the body's ability to fight cancer. Therefore, these medicines may be more appropriate for patients with inoperable advanced cancer, those in periods of chemotherapy intermission, or those during postoperative recovery. There has been an increased emphasis on such agents for prevention of cancer and inhibition of cancer metastasis. There has been an impressive renaissance in the search for semi-synthetic drugs or derivatives from natural compounds. Progress in this regard not only adds to the chemical bank but also leads to a better comprehension of the chemical basis of treatments lacking side effects for the treatment of cancers using drugs obtained from natural sources.

Further studies will be required to establish a strategy for basic molecular and clinical approaches for effective oral cancer therapy, which should be tailored to individual patients.

Conflict of interest

We have no financial relationships to disclose.

Author details

Masakatsu Fukuda* and Hideaki Sakashita

*Address all correspondence to: fukudam@dent.meikai.ac.jp

Division of Oral and Maxillofacial Surgery, Department of Diagnostic and Therapeutic Sciences, Meikai University School of Dentistry, Saitama, Japan

References

[1] Omran AR. The epidemiologic transition. A theory of the epidemiology of population change. The Milbank Memorial Fund Quarterly. 1971;**49**:509-538

[2] Gersten O, Wilmoth JR. The cancer transition in Japan since 1951. Demographic Research. 2002;**7**:271-306

[3] Bray F. Transitions in human development and the global cancer burden. In: Stewart BW, Wild CP, editors. World Cancer Report 2014. Lyon: IARC Press; 2014. pp. 42-55

[4] Maule M, Merletti F. Cancer transition and priorities for cancer control. The Lancet Oncology. 2012;**13**:745-746

[5] Parkin D, Bray F, Ferlay J, Pisani P. Global cancer statistics, 2001. CA: A Cancer Journal for Clinicians. 2005;**55**:74-108

[6] Argiris A, Karamouzis M, Raben D, Ferris R. Head and neck cancer. Lancet. 2008;**371**: 1695-1709

[7] Brandizz I, Gandolfo M, Velazco M, Cabrini R, Lanfranchi H. Clinical features and evolution of oral cancer, a study of 274 cases in Buenos Aires, Argentina. Medicina Oral, Patología Oral y Cirugía Bucal. 2008;**13**:E544-E5E8

[8] Stewart B, Greim H, Shuker D, Kauppinen T. Defence of IARC monographs. Lancet. 2003;**361**:13003-13006

[9] Xi S, Grandis J. Gene therapy for the treatment of oral squamous cell carcinoma. Journal of Dental Research. 2003;**82**:11-16

[10] Pereira M, Oliveira D, Landman G, Kowalski L. Histologic subtypes of oral squamous cell carcinoma: Prognostic relevance. Journal of the Canadian Dental Association. 2007;**73**:339-344

[11] Klein A. Parallel progression of primary tumours and metastases. Nature Reviews Cancer. 2009;**3**:302-312

[12] Fidler I. Critical factors in the biology of human cancer metastasis: Twenty-eighth GHA Clowes Memorial Award Lecture. Cancer Research. 1990;**50**:6130-6138

[13] Nguyen D, Massague J. Genetic determinants of cancer metastasis. Nature Reviews. Cancer. 2007;**8**:341-352

[14] Fidler I. Tumor heterogeneity and the biology of cancer invasion and metastasis. Cancer Research. 1978;**38**:2651-2660

[15] Mani SA, Guo W, Liao MJ, Eaton EN, Ayyanan A, Zhou AY, et al. The epithelial mesenchymal transition generates cells with properties of stem cells. Cell. 2008;**133**:704-715

[16] Barnhart B, Simon M. Metastasis and stem cells pathways. Cancer and Metastasis Reviews. 2007;**26**:261-271

[17] Freemont AJ, Hoyland JA. Cell adhesion molecules. Journal of Clinical Pathology Molecular Pathology. 1996;**49**:M321-M330

[18] Cyrus C, Jones EY. The molecular structure of cell adhesion molecules. Annual Review of Biochemistry. 1997;**66**:823-863

[19] Brackenbury R, Rutishauser U, Edelman GM. Distinct calcium-independent and calcium-dependent adhesion systems of chicken embryo cells. Proceedings of the National Academy of Sciences of the United States of America. 1981;**78**:387-391

[20] Lodish H, Berk A, Zipursky SL, Matsudaira P, Baltimore D, Darnell J. Cell-cell adhesion and communication. In: Molecular Cell Biology. 4th ed. New York: W. H. Freeman; 2000. Section 22.1

[21] Edelman GM, Crossin KL. Cell adhesion molecules: Implications for a molecular histology. Annual Review of Biochemistry. 1991;**60**:155-190

[22] He HT, Barbet J, Chaix JC, Goridis C. Phosphatidylinositol is involved in the membrane attachment of NCAM-120, the smallest component of the neural cell adhesion molecule. The EMBO Journal. 1986;**5**:2489-2494

[23] Nybrone O, Bock E. Structure and function of the neural cell adhesion molecules NCAM and L1. Advances in Experimental Medicine and Biology. 1990;**265**:185-196

[24] Barthels D, Vopper G, Boned A, Cremer H, Wille W. High degree of NCAM diversity generated by alternative RNA splicing in brain and muscle. The European Journal of Neuroscience. 1992;**4**:327-337

[25] Cunningham BA, Hoffman S, Rutishauser U, Hemperly JJ, Edelman GM. Molecular topography of the neural cell adhesion molecule NCAM: Surface orientation and location of sialic acid rich and binding regions. Proceedings of the National Academy of Sciences of the United States of America. 1983;**80**:3116-3120

[26] Gennarini G, Hirn M, Deagostini-Bazin H, Goridis C. Studies on the transmembrane disposition of the neural cell adhesion molecule N-CAM. The use of liposome-inserted radioiodinated N-CAM to study its transbilayer orientation. European Journal of Biochemistry. 1984;**142**:65-73

[27] Luo J, Miller MW. Transforming growth factor β1-regulated cell proliferation and expression of neural cell adhesion molecule in B104 neuroblastoma cells: Differential effects of ethanol. Journal of Neurochemistry. 1999;**72**:2286-2293

[28] Einheber S, Hannocks M-J, Metz CN, Rifkin DB, Salzer JL. Transforming growth factor-β1 regulates axon/Schwann cell interactions. The Journal of Cell Biology. 1995;**129**:443-458

[29] Stewart HJS, Rougon G, Dong Z, Dean C, Jessen KR, Mirsky R. TGF-βs upregulate NCAM and L1 expression in cultured Schwann cells, suppress cyclic AMP-induced expression of 04 and galactocerebroside, and are widely expressed in cells of the Schwann cell lineage *in vivo*. GLIA. 1995;**15**:419-436

[30] Seki H, Koyama K, Tanaka J, Sato Y, Umezawa A. Neural cell adhesion molecule and perineural invasion in gallbladder cancer. Journal of Surgical Oncology. 1995;**58**:97-100

[31] Seki H, Tanaka J, Sato Y, Kato Y, Umezawa A, Koyama K. Neural cell adhesion molecule (NCAM) and perineural invasion in bile duct cancer. Journal of Surgical Oncology. 1993;**53**:78-83

[32] Mooy CM, Luyten GP, de Jong PT, Jensen OA, Luider TM, van der Ham F, et al. Neural cell adhesion molecule distribution in primary and metastatic uveal melanoma. Human Pathology. 1995;**26**:1185-1190

[33] Gandour-Edwards R, Kapadia SB, Barnes L, Donald PJ, Janecka IP. Neural cell adhesion molecule in adenoid cystic carcinoma invading the skull base. Otolaryngology and Head and Neck Surgery. 1997;**117**:453-458

[34] Hutcheson JA, Vural E, Korourian S, Hanna E. Neural cell adhesion molecule expression in adenoid cystic carcinoma of the head and neck. Laryngoscope. 2000;**110**:946-948

[35] França CM, Jaeger MM, Jaeger RG, Araujo NS. The role of basement membrane proteins on the expression of neural cell adhesion molecule (N-CAM) in an adenoid cystic carcinoma cell line. Oral Oncology. 2000;**36**:248-252

[36] Fukuda M, Horiuchi Y, Oku Y, Ishikawa M, Suka N, Suzuki S, et al. Induction of apoptosis in human salivary gland tumor cells bv anti-NCAM antibody. Oncology Reports. 2005;**14**:1143-1149

[37] Sporns O, Edelman GM, Crossin KL. The neural cell adhesion molecule (NCAM) inhibits proliferation in primary cultures of rat astrocytes. Proceedings of the National Academy of Sciences of the United States of America. 1995;**92**:542-546

[38] Krushel LA, Sporns O, Cunningham BA, Crossin KL. Neural cell adhesion molecule (N-CAM) inhibits astrocyte proliferation after injury to different regions of the adult rat brain. Proceedings of the National Academy of Sciences of the United States of America. 1995;**92**:4323-4327

[39] Freston JW, Cimetidine I. Developments, pharmacology, and efficacy. Annals of Internal Medicine. 1982;**97**:573-580

[40] Adams WJ, Lawson JA, Morris DL. Cimetidine inhibits *in vivo* growth of human colon cancer and reverses histamine stimulated *in vitro* and *in vivo* growth. Gut. 1994;**35**:1632-1636

[41] Sasson AR, Gamagami R, An Z, Wang X, Moossa AR, Hoffman RM. Cimetidine: An inhibitor or promoter of tumor growth? International Journal of Cancer. 1999;**81**:835-838

[42] Lawson JA, Adams WJ, Morris DL. Ranitidine and cimetidine differ in their *in vitro* and *in vivo* effects on human colonic cancer growth. British Journal of Cancer. 1996;**73**:872-876

[43] Reynolds JL, Akhter J, Morris DL. *In vitro* effect of histamine and histamine HI and H2 receptor antagonists on cellular proliferation of human malignant melanoma cell lines. Melanoma Research. 1996;**6**:95-99

[44] Lefranc F, Yeaton P, Brotchi J, Kiss R. Cimetidine, an unexpected anti-tumor agent, and its potential for the treatment of glioblastoma. International Journal of Oncology. 2006;**28**:1021-1030

[45] Fukuda M, Kusama K, Sakashita H. Cimetidine inhibits salivary gland tumor cell adhesion to neural cells and induces apoptosis by blocking NCAM expression. BMC Cancer. 2008;**8**:376. DOI: 10.1186/1471-2407-8-376

[46] Bergelson JM, Cunningham JA, Droguett G, Kurt-Jones EA, Krithivas A, Hong JS, et al. Isolation of a common receptor for Coxsackie B viruses and adenoviruses 2 and 5. Science. 1997;**275**:1320-1323

[47] Cohen CJ, Shieh JT, Pickles RJ, Okegawa T, Hsieh JT, Bergelson JM. The coxsackievirus and adenovirus receptor is a transmembrane component of the tight junction. Proceedings of the National Academy of Sciences of the United States of America. 2001;**98**:15191-15196

[48] Sollerbrant K, Raschperger E, Mirza M, Engstrom U, Philipson L, Ljungdahl PO, et al. The coxsackievirus and adenovirus receptor (CAR) forms a complex with the PDZ domain-containing protein ligand of numb protein-X (LNX). The Journal of Biological Chemistry. 2003;**278**:7439-7444

[49] Coyne CB, Voelker T, Pichla SL, Bergelson JM. The coxsackievirus and adenovirus receptor interacts with the multi-PDZ domain protein-1 (MUPP-1) within the tight junction. The Journal of Biological Chemistry. 2004;**279**:48079-48084

[50] Excoffon KJ, Hruska-Hageman A, Klotz M, Traver GL, Zabner J. A role for the PDZ-binding domain of the coxsackie B virus and adenovirus receptor (CAR) in cell adhesion and growth. Journal of Cell Science. 2004;**117**:4401-4409

[51] Mirza M, Raschperger E, Philipson L, Pettersson RF, Sollerbrant K. The cell surface protein coxsackie- and adenovirus receptor (CAR) directly associates with the ligand-of-numb protein-X2 (LNX2). Experimental Cell Research. 2005;**309**:110-120

[52] Raschperger E, Thyberg J, Pettersson S, Philipson L, Fuxe J, Pettersson RF. The coxsackie- and adenovirus receptor (CAR) is an *in vivo* marker for epithelial tight junctions, with

a potential role in regulating permeability and tissue homeostasis. Experimental Cell Research. 2006;**312**:1566-1580

[53] Okegawa T, Li Y, Pong RC, Bergelson JM, Zhou J, Hsieh JT. The dual impact of coxsackie and adenovirus receptor expression on human prostate cancer gene therapy. Cancer Research. 2000;**60**:5031-5036

[54] Bruning A, Runnebaum IB. CAR is a cell-cell adhesion protein in human cancer cells and is expressionally modulated by dexamethasone, TNFalpha, and TGFbeta. Gene Therapy. 2003;**10**:198-205

[55] Rauen KA, Sudilovsky D, Le JL, Chew KL, Hann B, Weinberg V, et al. Expression of the coxsackie adenovirus receptor in normal prostate and in primary and metastatic prostate carcinoma: Potential relevance to gene therapy. Cancer Research. 2002;**62**:3812-3818

[56] Sachs MD, Rauen KA, Ramamurthy M, Dodson JL, De Marzo AM, Putzi MJ, et al. Integrin alpha(v) and coxsackie adenovirus receptor expression in clinical bladder cancer. Urology. 2002;**60**:531-536

[57] Matsumoto K, Shariat SF, Ayala GE, Rauen KA, Lerner SP. Loss of coxsackie and adenovirus receptor expression is associated with features of aggressive bladder cancer. Urology. 2005;**66**:441-446

[58] Korn WM, Macal M, Christian C, Lacher MD, McMillan A, Rauen KA, et al. Expression of the coxsackievirus- and adenovirus receptor in gastrointestinal cancer correlates with tumor differentiation. Cancer Gene Therapy. 2006;**13**:792-797

[59] Pitti RM, Marsters SA, Ruppert S, Donahue CJ, Moore A, Ashkenazi A. Induction of apoptosis by Apo-2 ligand, a new member of the tumor necrosis factor cytokine family. The Journal of Biological Chemistry. 1996;**271**:12687-12690

[60] Wiley SR, Schooley K, Smolak PJ, Din WS, Huang CP, Nicholl JK, et al. Identification and characterization of a new member of the TNF family that induces apoptosis. Immunity. 1995;**3**:673-682

[61] Nagata S. Apoptosis by death factor. Cell. 1997;**88**:355-365

[62] Nakashima M, Sonoda K, Watanabe T. Inhibition of cell growth and induction of apoptotic cell death by the human tumor-associated antigen RCAS1. Nature Medicine. 1999;**5**:938-942

[63] Degli-Esposti MA, Smolak PJ, Walczak H, Waugh J, Huang CP, RF DB, et al. Cloning and characterization of TRAIL-R3, a novel member of the emerging TRAIL receptor family. The Journal of Experimental Medicine. 1997;**186**:1165-1170

[64] Pan G, Ni J, Wei YF, Yu G, Gentz R, Dixit VM. An antagonist decoy receptor and a death domain-containing receptor for TRAIL. Science. 1997;**277**:815-818

[65] Sheridan JP, Marsters SA, Pitti RM, Gurney A, Skubatch M, Baldwin D, et al. Control of TRAIL-induced apoptosis by a family of signaling and decoy receptors. Science. 1997;**277**:818-821

[66] Marsters SA, Sheridan JP, Pitti RM, Huang A, Skubatch M, Baldwin D, et al. A novel receptor for Apo2L/TRAIL contains a truncated death domain. Current Biology. 1997;**7**: 1003-1006

[67] Pan G, Ni J, Yu G, Wei YF, Dixit VM. TRUNDD, a new member of the TRAIL receptor family that antagonizes TRAIL signaling. FEBS Letters. 1998;**424**:41-45

[68] Griffith TS, Rauch CT, Smolak PJ, Waugh JY, Boiani N, Lynch DH, et al. Functional analysis of TRAIL receptors using monoclonal antibodies. Journal of Immunology. 1999;**162**:2597-2605

[69] Rieger J, Naumann U, Glaser T, Ashkenazi A, Weller M. APO2 ligand: A novel lethal weapon against malignant glioma? FEBS Letters. 1998;**427**:124-128

[70] Marsters SA, Pitti RM, Donahue CJ, Ruppert S, Bauer KD, Ashkenazi A. Activation of apoptosis by Apo-2 ligand is independent of FADD but blocked by CrmA. Current Biology. 1996;**6**:750-752

[71] Fukuda M, Hamao A, Tanaka A, Kitada M, Suzuki S, Kusama K, et al. Tumor necrosis factor-related apoptosis-inducing ligand (TRAIL/APO2L) and its receptors expression in human squamous cell carcinoma of the oral cavity. Oncology Reports. 2003;**10**:1113-1119

[72] Strand S, Hofmann WJ, Hug H, Muller M, Otto G, Stramd D, et al. Lymphocyte apoptosis induced by CD95 (APO-1/Fas) ligand- expressing tumor cells: A mechanism of immune evasion? Nature Medicine. 1996;**2**:1361-1366

[73] Hahne M, Rimoldi D, Schroter M, Romero P, Schreier M, French LE, et al. Melanoma cell expression of Fas (Apo-1/CD95) ligand: Implications for tumor immune escape. Science (Washington, DC). 1996;**274**:1363-1366

[74] Gratas C, Tohma Y, Barnas C, Taniere P, Hainaut P, Ohgaki H. Up-regulation of Fas (APO-1/CD95) ligand and down-regulation of Fas expression in human esophageal cancer. Cancer Research. 1998;**58**:2057-2062

[75] Keane MM, Ettenberg SA, Nau MM, Russell EK, Lipkowitz S. Chemotherapy augments TRAIL-induced apoptosis in breast cell lines. Cancer Research. 1999;**59**:734-741

[76] Wen J, Ramadevi N, Nguyen D, Perkins C, Worthington E, Bhalla K. Antileukemic drugs increase death receptor 5 levels and enhance Apo-2L-induced apoptosis of human acute leukemia cells. Blood. 2000;**96**:3900-3906

[77] Knight MJ, Riffkin CD, Muscat AM, Ashley DM, Hawkins CJ. Analysis of FasL and TRAIL induced apoptosis pathways in glioma cells. Oncogene. 2001;**20**:5789-5798

[78] Pai SI, Wu GS, Özören N, Wu L, Jen J, Sidransky D, et al. Rare loss-of-function mutation of a death receptor gene in head and neck cancer. Cancer Research. 1998;**58**:3513-3518

[79] Fisher MJ, Virmani AK, Wu L, Aplenc R, Harper JC, Powell SM, et al. Nucleotide substitution in the Ectodomain of TRAIL receptor DR4 is associated with lung cancer and head and neck cancer. Clinical Cancer Research. 2001;**7**:1688-1697

[80] Scaffidi C, Kirchhoff S, Krammer PH, Peter ME. Apoptosis signaling in lymphocytes. Current Opinion in Immunology. 1999;**11**:277-285

[81] Nakamura M, Rieger J, Weller M, Kim J, Kleihues P, Ohgaki H. APO2L/TRAIL expression in human brain tumors. Acta Neuropathologica. 2000;**99**:1-6

[82] Matsuzaki H, Schmied BM, Ulrich A, Standop J, Schneider MB, Batra SK, et al. Combination of tumor necrosis factor-related apoptosis-inducing ligand (TRAIL) and actinomycin D induces apoptosis even in TRAIL-resistant human pancreatic cancer cells. Clinical Cancer Research. 2001;**7**:407-414

[83] Mitsiades CS, Treon SP, Mitsiades N, Shima Y, Richardson P, Schlossman R, et al. Apo2L ligand selectively induces apoptosis and overcomes drug resistance in multiple myeloma: Therapeutic applications. Blood. 2001;**98**:795-804

[84] Fukuda M, Sakashita H, Hayashi H, Shiono J, Miyake G, Komine Y, et al. Synergism between α-mangostin and TRAIL induces apoptosis in squamous cell carcinoma of the oral cavity through the mitochondrial pathway. Oncology Reports. 2017;**38**:3439-3446

[85] Joffre C, Barrow R, Menard L, Calleja V, Hart IR, Kermorgant S. A direct role for Met endocytosis in tumorigenesis. Nature Cell Biology. 2011;**13**:827-837

[86] Maina F, Panté G, Helmbacher F, Andres R, Porthin A, Davies AM, et al. Coupling Met to specific pathways results in distinct developmental outcomes. Molecular Cell. 2001;**7**:1293-1306

[87] Gentile A, Trusolino L, Comoglio PM. The Met tyrosine kinase receptor in development and cancer. Cancer Metastasis Reviews. 2008;**27**:85-94

[88] Chu SH, Feng DF, Zhang H, Chen ET, Duan ZX, Li XY, et al. c-Met-targeted RNA interference inhibits growth and metastasis of glioma U251 cells *in vitro*. Journal of Neuro-Oncology. 2009;**93**:183-189

[89] Merlin S, Pietronave S, Locarno D, Valente G, Follenzi A, Prat M. Deletion of the ectodomain unleashes the transforming, invasive, and tumorigenic potential of the MET oncogene. Cancer Science. 2009;**100**:633-638

[90] Birchmeier C, Birchmeier W, Gherardi E, Vande Woude GF. Met, metastasis, motility and more. Nature Reviews. Molecular Cell Biology. 2003;**4**:915-925

[91] You WK, DM MD. The hepatocyte growth factor/c-Met signaling pathway as a therapeutic target to inhibit angiogenesis. BMB Reports. 2008;**41**:833-839

[92] Kentsis A, Reed C, Rice KL, Sanda T, Rodig SJ, Tholouli E, et al. Autocrine activation of the MET receptor tyrosine kinase in acute myeloid leukemia. Nature Medicine. 2012;**18**:1118-1122

[93] Graziano F, Galluccio N, Lorenzini P, Ruzzo A, Canestrari E, D'Emidio S, et al. Genetic activation of the MET pathway and prognosis of patients with high-risk, radically resected gastric cancer. Journal of Clinical Oncology. 2011;**29**(36):4789-4795

[94] Peters S, Adjei AA. MET: A promising anticancer therapeutic target. Nature Reviews. Clinical Oncology. 2012;**9**:314-326

[95] Sun S, Wang Z. Head neck squamous cell carcinoma c-Met (+) cells display cancer stem cell properties and are responsible for cisplatin-resistance and metastasis. International Journal of Cancer. 2011;**129**:2337-2348

[96] Lo Muzio L, Farina A, Rubini C, Coccia E, Capogreco M, Colella G, et al. Effect of c-Met expression on survival in head and neck squamous cell carcinoma. Tumour Biology. 2006;**27**(3):115-121

[97] Ainscow EK, Brand MD. Top-down control analysis of ATP turnover, glycolysis and oxidative phosphorylation in rat hepatocytes. European Journal of Biochemistry. 1999;**263**:671-685

[98] Lopez-Lazaro M. The Warburg effect: Why and how do cancer cells activate glycolysis in the presence of oxygen? Anti-Cancer Agents in Medicinal Chemistry. 2008;**8**:305-312

[99] Warburg O. On the origin of cancer cells. Science. 1956;**123**:309-314

[100] Warburg O. On respiratory impairment in cancer cells. Science. 1956;**124**:269-270

[101] Ward PS, Thompson CB. Metabolic reprogramming: A cancer hallmark even warburg did not anticipate. Cancer Cell. 2012;**21**:297-308

[102] Koppenol WH, Bounds PL, Dang CV. Otto Warburg's contributions to current concepts of cancer metabolism. Nature Reviews. Cancer. 2011;**11**:325-337

[103] Lunt SY, Vander Heiden MG. Aerobic glycolysis: Meeting the metabolic requirements of cell proliferation. Annual Review of Cell and Developmental Biology. 2011;**27**:441-464

[104] Dang CV, Semenza GL. Oncogenic alterations of metabolism. Trends in Biochemical Sciences. 1999;**24**:68-72

[105] Semenza GL. Defining the role of hypoxia-inducible factor 1 in cancer biology and therapeutics. Oncogene. 2010;**29**:625-634

[106] Gordan JD, Thompson CB, Simon MC. HIF and c-Myc: Sibling rivals for control of cancer cell metabolism and proliferation. Cancer Cell. 2007;**12**:108-113

[107] Gleadle JM, Ratcliffe PJ. Induction of hypoxia-inducible factor-1, erythropoietin, vascular endothelial growth factor, and glucose transporter-1 by hypoxia: Evidence against a regulatory role for Src kinase. Blood. 1997;**89**:503-509

[108] Fukuda M, Ohmori Y, Sakashita H. In: Biswas S, editor. Tumor Microenvironment and Myelomonocytic Cells. IntechOpen Limited; 2012. pp. 201-208. DOI: 10.5772/1507

[109] Maxfield FR. Plasma membrane microdomains. Current Opinion in Cell Biology. 2002;**14**:483-487

[110] Mukherjee S, Maxfield FR. Membrane domains. Annual Review of Cell and Developmental Biology. 2004;**20**:839-866

[111] Pomorski T, Hrafnsdottir S, Devaux PF, van Meer G. Lipid distribution and transport across cellular membranes. Seminars in Cell & Developmental Biology. 2001;**12**:139-148

[112] Van Meer G. Membranes in motion. EMBO Reports. 2010;**11**:331-333

[113] Van Meer G, Voelker DR, Feigenson GW. Membrane lipids: Where they are and how they behave. Nature Reviews. Molecular Cell Biology. 2008;**9**:112-124

[114] Guo D, Bell EH, Chakravarti A. Lipid metabolism emerges as a promising target for malignant glioma therapy. CNS Oncology. 2013;**2**:289-299

[115] Menendez JA, Lupu R. Fatty acid synthase and the lipogenic phenotype in cancer pathogenesis. Nature Reviews. Cancer. 2007;**7**:763-777

[116] Zechner R, Strauss JG, Haemmerle G, Lass A, Zimmermann R. Lipolysis: Pathway under construction. Current Opinion in Lipidology. 2005;**16**:333-340

[117] Abramson HN. The lipogenesis pathway as a cancer target. Journal of Medicinal Chemistry. 2011;**54**:5615-5638

[118] Grossi-Paoletti E, Paoletti P, Fumagalli R. Lipids in brain tumors. Journal of Neurosurgery. 1971;**34**:454-455

[119] Podo F. Tumour phospholipid metabolism. NMR in Biomedicine. 1999;**12**:413-439

[120] Santos CR, Schulze A. Lipid metabolism in cancer. The FEBS Journal. 2012;**279**:2610-2623

[121] Yoon S, Lee MY, Park SW, Moon JS, Koh YK, Ahn YH, et al. Up-regulation of acetyl-CoA carboxylase alpha and fatty acid synthase by human epidermal growth factor receptor 2 at the translational level in breast cancer cells. The Journal of Biological Chemistry. 2007;**282**:26122-26131

[122] Weiss L, Hoffmann GE, Schreiber R, Andres H, Fuchs E, Korber E, et al. Fatty-acid biosynthesis in man, a pathway of minor importance. Purification, optimal assay conditions, and organ distribution of fatty-acid synthase. Biological Chemistry Hoppe-Seyler. 1986;**367**:905-912

[123] Migita T, Ruiz S, Fornari A, Fiorentino M, Priolo C, Zadra G, et al. Fatty acid synthase: A metabolic enzyme and candidate oncogene in prostate cancer. Journal of the National Cancer Institute. 2009;**101**:519-532

[124] Carvalho MA, Zecchin KG, Seguin F, Bastos DC, Agostini M, Rangel ALCA, et al. Fatty acid synthase inhibition with orlistat promotes apoptosis and reduces cell growth and lymph node metastasis in a mouse melanoma model. International Journal of Cancer. 2008;**123**:2557-2565

[125] Rohr-Udilova N, Bauer E, Timelthaler G, Eferl R, Stolze K, Pinter M, et al. Impact of glutathione peroxidase 4 on cell proliferation, angiogenesis and cytokine production in hepatocellular carcinoma. Oncotarget. 2018;**9**:10054-10068

[126] Cao JY, Dixon SJ. Mechanisms of ferroptosis. Cellular and Molecular Life Sciences. 2016;**73**:2195-2209